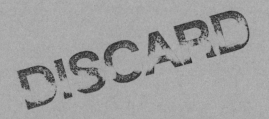

# Romance Rehab

# Romance Rehab

## 10 Steps to Rescue Your Relationship

By Dr. Jan Hoistad

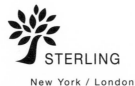

STERLING

New York / London
www.sterlingpublishing.com

STERLING and the distinctive Sterling logo are registered trademarks of Sterling Publishing Co., Inc.

**Library of Congress Cataloging-in-Publication Data**

Hoistad, Jan.
   Romance rehab : 10 steps to rescue your relationship / by Jan Hoistad.
      p. cm.
   Includes bibliographical references and index.
   ISBN 978-1-4027-6548-3
   1. Couples therapy. 2. Marital psychotherapy. I. Title.
   RC488.5.H613 2010
   616.89'1562--dc22

                                                                    2009026298


                           2  4  6  8  10 9  7  5  3  1

                    Published by Sterling Publishing Co., Inc.
                    387 Park Avenue South, New York, NY 10016
                            © 2010 by Jan Hoistad
                    Distributed in Canada by Sterling Publishing
                   c/o Canadian Manda Group, 165 Dufferin Street
                          Toronto, Ontario, Canada M6K 3H6
            Distributed in the United Kingdom by GMC Distribution Services
         Castle Place, 166 High Street, Lewes, East Sussex, England BN7 1XU
             Distributed in Australia by Capricorn Link (Australia) Pty. Ltd.
                       P.O. Box 704, Windsor, NSW 2756, Australia

                       Sterling ISBN 978-1-4027-6548-3

          For information about custom editions, special sales, premium and
            corporate purchases, please contact Sterling Special Sales
          Department at 800-805-5489 or specialsales@sterlingpublishing.com.

# Contents

*For Megan, Mac, and the promise of healthy future generations.*

## Introduction

# The Secret of Lasting Love: Your Big Picture Adventure

No one is born knowing how to have a healthy, mutually satisfying relationship. However, you can learn how to create the partnership you've always hoped for. If you think your romance needs rehab, this book will show you a solution. If your relationship is on the verge of a breakdown, *Romance Rehab* can help. If you want to take your basically healthy partnership to a new level or make sure your new relationship is off to a rock-solid start, discover the art of Big Picture Partnering to learn the secrets of lasting love.

*Romance Rehab* teaches you the 10 Steps of Big Picture Partnering. What is Big Picture Partnering? It's a new way of looking at relationships. It is what you need to create a partnership that is consistently nourishing, affirming, and downright wonderful. It means creating a relationship that stays strong because both of you are getting what you want most in your lives and consistently creating and living your dreams together.

If you were asked to describe the Big Picture of your relationship with your spouse or partner right now, which would be closest to your reaction?

- Your heart flutters with excitement at the thought of your newfound love and your dreams and hopes together.

- You pause and feel the warmth you have for your partner—warmth that often becomes buried under piles of laundry or stacks of bills but quickly surfaces again given the opportunity.

- You yearn for some time and freedom to be alone with your partner—away from the kids and your careers and the endless responsibilities that have taken over much of your lives.

- You've been fighting or avoiding each other—so many topics are unresolved and the resentment is growing—you are tired of the discord and wonder how you will get the closeness back.

- You remember the dreams the two of you had talked about accomplishing together but have never been able to attain.

- You remember the way you felt long ago, when you and your partner first fell in love—and you wonder how so many of those feelings have disappeared over the years.

- You feel both frightened and hopeful—hopeful because after a string of poor decisions about partners, you've finally committed yourself to someone wonderful but frightened that you may make the same mistakes all over again.

- You wonder, now that the kids are finally grown or because you're nearing retirement, if the two of you can renew the passion and commitment you felt for each other so many years ago.

If any of these feelings resonate with you, welcome. You've come to the right place. *Romance Rehab* will guide you through the 10-Step approach of Big Picture Partnering, a program that helps couples rescue or rejuvenate their romance and create a new and ongoing relationship based on commitment, support, adventure, and joy.

We all know the attraction, excitement, and understanding that accompany the early days and months of courtship. This initial connection often wanes as we take each other and our relationship for granted. After we've been together for a time, we often feel as though our friends and colleagues treat us better than our closest loved one does. How can we keep the good feelings alive or reinvigorate them if they have diminished? *Romance Rehab* will show you how.

In this day and age, with so many choices, relationships are more confusing than ever. We are also living so much longer that finding ways to keep love alive is challenging for everyone. There is no one formula for a healthy, satisfying relationship anymore. Years ago (in your grandparents' and great-grandparents' day) when there were fewer options, people knew what was expected of them and of a relationship. They did not question their happiness or satisfaction as we do today. They often married, sometimes for love, but almost always for survival and economic reasons.

All that has changed. We want and expect so much more. We want to be fulfilled as individuals, and we want to love and be loved, to be happy in our most important relationship.

*Romance Rehab* offers a new model. In this easy to follow program, you will learn the concepts, tools, and skills that help you create a satisfying partnership *together*—a partnership that is as satisfying as your work, your friendships, and your hobbies. *Romance Rehab* will teach you how to put things right when they have gotten off track. Big Picture Partnering is the solution. It isn't just a skill or technique, neither is it therapy or fixing what's wrong with either partner in the relationship. *Romance Rehab* teaches you the 10 Steps that, when combined and practiced consistently, keep your connection alive and your relationship rock-solid. This Big Picture approach is a completely different way of being in a partnership—and of being together in the world—that offers couples lives full of spontaneity and possibility.

I've been showing couples how to rehab their romance through Big Picture Partnering for more than twenty years, both in workshops and in counseling and coaching sessions. I've watched couples use this 10-Step approach to blossom together, to deepen their commitment to each other, and to build the lives they most want to lead jointly.

## How to Use This Book

*Romance Rehab* will lead you through a process that teaches both you and your partner the 10 Steps of successful partnering. These 10 Steps will help you clarify your values, communicate more effectively, and resolve disagreements that have diminished your relationship energy. By applying the 10 Steps, you will find renewed commitment and vitality to help you accomplish your Big Picture goals together, dream together, and then turn those dreams into reality—day by day, year by year. Big Picture Partnering shows you how to synchronize yourselves into a true partnership without giving away any of your individuality or freedom.

If you've been fighting, I will ask you to stop for now while you learn new ways to communicate and interact. Then you will revisit your differences and have the tools to find win/win solutions. If you haven't been fighting, but issues have been swept under the rug or you want to make your relationship even better, the Big Picture Partnering approach offers you the skills to accomplish these goals.

The 10 Steps to successful partnering can even work if your partner doesn't want to undertake the program with you. As you complete the exercises in the book, you can clarify your own issues while starting conversations with your partner that will help your partnership evolve.

Big Picture Partnering can provide answers for adults of any age, from young couples to couples well into retirement. It doesn't matter what gender you or your partner are, what religion you do or don't practice, or whether you and your partner are married. All you need is an honest and earnest commitment to each other and a desire to live a full, joyous life together.

If your romance needs rehab, if you yearn for a partnership that will nourish, support, and delight you—keep reading. You can look forward to a partnership that enriches, empowers, and enlivens you both for a lifetime.

# Where Is Your Relationship Now?

You have picked up *Romance Rehab* because you want to change or improve your relationship. In order to make a change, you need to know your starting point. You need to identify what kind of relationship you have now. You also must know the destination—or type of relationship—you most desire.

In Part I of *Romance Rehab* you will be introduced to three different common ways that couples relate. These are the Traditional, Merged, and Roommate styles. You'll learn how each approach may work for a time, but how they can also lead to discontent and dissatisfaction. Then you'll be introduced to the Big Picture Partnering Style and its benefits. Throughout this section, you'll be guided to reflect on your current relationship mode—and how you'd really like it to be.

From this "Big Picture" understanding, in Part II of *Romance Rehab* you'll work through the 10 Steps to create the change you most desire.

## Chapter 1

# Discover Your Relationship Style

In this chapter and the next, you are going to consider four relationship styles:

- Traditional

- Merged

- Roommate

- Big Picture Partnering

As we explore each relationship style, we will pay particular attention to the four dimensions in which that style

1. promotes healthy development of each person's full, mature self—the individual's independence and uniqueness, as well as the couple's healthy interdependence in which they come together in equal and mutually satisfying ways;

2. provides opportunities for individual as well as mutual pursuits;

3. approaches decision making;

4. offers consistent opportunities for intimacy building and emotional connection.

3

Because no one is born knowing how to have a relationship, you unconsciously look to the role models in your lives for examples. Typically, you absorbed the examples of your parents and other adults around you in your growing-up years, even if you were unaware of doing so. This is what makes them unconscious. You may also have looked to role models as you entered college or the work force, developing adult friendships and observing other relationships and marriages.

When push comes to shove, however, the behaviors and communication styles you observed in your childhood relationships are the behaviors and communication styles you revert to until you consciously

- reflect on your relating style;

- make decisions to keep what is working and discard what is not working;

- learn new ways to interact and communicate that are healthy and more compatible with the relationship you want to achieve;

- work together toward instilling the new ways as lifelong habits.

With so many relationship options and little direction about what makes a good relationship, couples often work at cross-purposes. Like you, they may find that their relationship feels good only some of the time. Wouldn't it be nice to know how to keep it feeling good and working well most of the time? By learning about these four relating styles you will become empowered to make skillful choices about the kind of relationship you want to have.

As you read, you may recognize some aspects of each style in your relationship. Most couples start with a combination of styles. When a mixture of styles exists, partners are often confused, because one person may be operating under one set of assumptions, and the other person may unconsciously switch to another style and set of assumptions.

While every couple consciously or unconsciously chooses the kind of relationship they want to create, in my work with couples over the past thirty years, 100 percent of couples who come to me desire a Big Picture Partnership once the partners understand these four different styles of relating. They would not have used that term before learning about the four styles; nor do they have all the tools necessary to build a Big Picture Partnership until they learn the approach. However, as they study the Traditional, Merged, and Roommate styles and reflect on their desires, couples observe that aspects of each feel OK sometimes but are not ultimately fulfilling in a lasting

## ✚ REHAB TOOLKIT
### How Are We Doing?

Stop and individually reflect on your relationship for a moment. Have your notebook and a pen handy. You will want to jot down some thoughts you have before you learn more about the four styles. You will expand on these thoughts in the individual and couple exercises at the end of this chapter. Ask yourself these questions:

- "How do I know my partnership is going well? What are the signs I am aware of?" (Some questions to guide you are, "How do I feel? How does my partner treat me? How do I treat my partner? What am I thinking about? What is my energy like? What kind of activities do I engage in individually and with my partner? Typically, how long are the periods when things are going well?")

- "How do I know when my partnership is not going well? What are the signs?" Use the questions above to guide your responses.

- Are you aware of what happens when you go from relating well to relating poorly? Identify what happens as clearly and specifically as you can.

- How do the two of you get stuck? How do you contribute to the two of you getting stuck? How do you contribute to the two of you staying stuck?

- List five things that usually help to put your relationship back on track. How often do you remember to perform these five things? If you don't accomplish them, what stops you from doing so?

relationship. They learn, as you will, that Big Picture Partnering offers an approach that makes their relationship long lasting—and fulfilling—every day and at every step along the way.

Let's look at all four styles. They form a backdrop from which you can choose how you build your most intimate relationship.

## The Traditional Style

The first way of relating is the one most likely modeled by your parents or grandparents: the Traditional Style. This style has been the norm in marriages for many generations and across many cultures. You may recognize aspects of this style in your own relationship.

Simply illustrated, the Traditional Style might look like this:

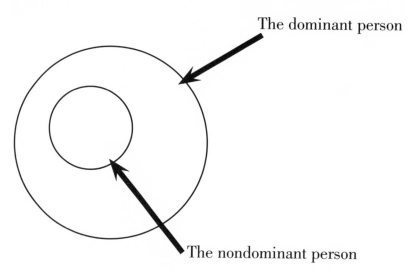

The dominant person

The nondominant person

*In the Traditional Style of relationship, one person has more power, especially in decision making.*

In the Traditional Style, one person has more decision-making power than the other. This does not necessarily mean that the dominant partner misuses or abuses his or her power. What it does mean is that one person in the couple usually makes the ultimate decisions. The male or female may take on this dominant role because the couple has assigned this person the decision-making authority or because one partner is more forceful, the other more passive. In the past, the man often assumed the dominant decision-making role, simply because both partners followed tradition. Sometimes the man wields decision-making power over more worldly aspects such as finances, and the woman makes most of the decisions about the home, child-rearing, and social activities.

If you evaluate your style as Traditional, use the four dimensions on page 3 to assess whether the style is chosen consciously, as a healthy combination of interdependence and independence, or whether one or both of you are simply avoiding making decisions or conflict by allowing your partner to take the lead. This approach would stifle your individual healthy growth. It would also limit intimacy-building and emotional connection because you are not sharing your true self.

Whether the people within a Traditional relationship promote independence and interdependence is determined by each couple. Sometimes a Traditional couple will do most things independently. He goes to work and hangs out with the guys; she raises the children and has her work and hobbies and friendship activities. They may come together around dinnertime, religious activities, some social engagements, and children's after-school events.

Some Traditional couples are very emotionally connected. Others do not know each other much at all. They choose to continue their Traditional Style because they may not wish to reveal themselves, or they may not wish to perform the work becoming close sometimes takes.

## Intimacy and Emotional Connection

Intimacy is getting to know someone who is different from you, then making space for those differences and accommodating those unique qualities in a relationship. It doesn't mean you have to like everything your partner does or necessarily agree on everything. Rather it is a nonjudgmental caring, a desire to know another person that develops out of a sense of openness and curiosity about that person, how he or she experiences life, what he or she values, enjoys, desires. It is also the willingness to share the same about you.

Intimacy is not just a feeling of being "in love." It is a combination of care, respect, wanting to know your partner's thoughts, feelings, and desires, and a willingness to work together to meet some of those.

Getting to know someone too quickly is not necessarily intimacy. It may simply be an emotional sharing that makes you feel connected for a brief time. True intimacy develops over time: It is the knowledge that we are willing to "know" each other, and continue getting to know each other, and that knowing is an evolving, growing, lifetime event.

When you are a couple for a long time, intimacy includes balancing acceptance of another and yourself with challenging each other to grow or develop more fully. Sometimes it is a feeling; often it is an action involving respect, caring, deep understanding, and acceptance, along with interactions and communication that promote mutual growth.

The feeling of safety with that person, the feeling of being cared about, accepted, not judged, and the feeling of being on the same team is what we call emotional connection. You can feel emotionally connected in the same room, while you are each off at work, or when you are across the globe.

Many Traditional couples report satisfying relationships, and some point out that it results in successfully circumventing potential power struggles and conflicts. Some even feel it is a God-given preference. The Traditional Style can spell out roles and tasks very clearly when there are young children to raise or when one person has the main breadwinning function and is on a career path that requires intense involvement.

You might know a couple like Al and Sharon, who exemplify the Traditional Style. Al is a high-level vice president at a Midwestern company. He comes from a culture of 1950s-style family values. He and Sharon are in their early thirties, with three children under the age of nine. Sharon is a stay-at-home mom and a stand-by-your-man kind of woman. She never questions Al's work choices, including their frequent job-related moves. She and the kids have had a hard time making long-term friendships. She hopes they stay in their current town until the kids have grown, but that decision will be left to Al. Sharon is proud to be at Al's side at church and at community and social events. They are both pleased with her role as Al's wife, and with her skills as a homemaker. She has dinner on the table at seven, shortly after Al arrives home from the office. If they have plans to go out for the evening, Sharon will have made arrangements for the sitter. Al spends time with the children after dinner until Sharon takes over and gets them ready for bed.

Sharon and Al came to see me because their relationship was feeling routine and Sharon didn't know why she was dissatisfied. I became concerned that their relationship did not make room for individual growth. I wondered if they could accommodate the conversations, openness to hearing each other's dissatisfactions, and change that are hallmarks of true intimacy. Al seemed content with the way things were going, and I wasn't sure he was concerned about Sharon's growing dissatisfaction.

The opportunity for connection and intimacy building in the Traditional Style is dependent upon the choices, needs, and desires of the person with the most power. When that person, usually the husband, feels that time with his partner is important and valuable, then talking, affection, and sex may occur on a regular and mutually fulfilling basis.

If, however, the dominant person is out of touch with the other person's needs, or simply doesn't think those needs are important, then connection and intimacy is missing.

## In the Traditional Style

One member of the pair is dominant and makes the ultimate decisions for both partners. One may be foremost in all aspects of life or may take over leading in certain aspects of life. In the Traditional Style, the emotional connection and opportunities for intimacy building vary for each couple because the degree of closeness and sharing is dependent on the desires and expectations of the person who is more dominant.

## The Merged Style

In the Merged Style of relating, individuals have few personal boundaries and little autonomy. They think, feel, and act interdependently in most areas of their life. They sometimes appear interchangeable in their thoughts, feelings, interests, and desires. Many couples have some Merged qualities; I have worked with only two who were Merged in many ways. In one circumstance, the woman wanted to grow; in the other, both partners realized they needed a more mature relationship. I think seeing Merged couples in therapy is probably rare because fully Merged couples seldom seek outside help as they are so self-contained. What is important is for you to identify small ways in which you may be Merged in your relating style and to determine if these ways of relating are right for you.

As the diagram below shows, the fully Merged couple shares the same psychological, mental, and emotional space:

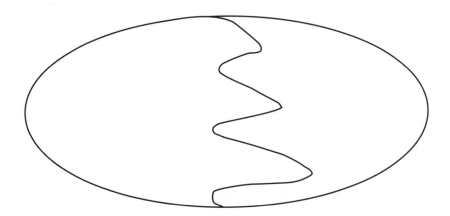

*In the Merged Style of relationship, two people are halves of a whole—codependent, interdependent, and interchangeable in thoughts, feelings, interests, and desires.*

Decision making for a Merged couple appears seamless. They go along with each other because they seldom do or decide anything that would be surprising or unusual. Typically, they stick to prescribed and expected choices, decisions, and responses, and they know exactly what to expect from each other. Often the person who is the least passive at that moment voices a preference, and the partner just goes along. Sometimes this is because one or both feel they cannot say what they want so they give in to their partner; sometimes it is because striking out independently causes their partner to become angry or unhappy or to feel betrayed. From a mental-health perspective, this style is not good for individual development.

Merging results in codependent and caretaking behavior. Individuality is sacrificed in always doing what others want—or what you surmise others want of you. Examples include a person who never offers an idea about what to do on a date; or someone who is always rubbing your back or getting you a cup of tea, even when you may not want one. That partner may want the back rub or the cup of tea and unconsciously hopes you will know this and return the favor. Sometimes people call this being "nice," but when it is overdone, one individual sacrifices self, needs, wants, and desires for the other.

When you're around such couples, you might notice that they may finish each other's thoughts—not just sentences—and have such a uniform point of view that they seem to have little individuality. Their closeness may appear as intimacy, while their responses or thoughts may seem rote, rigid, and routine. They are often inseparable, sometimes in an almost charming way, as in very old couples who have been together for fifty or sixty years. However, when one partner is away, the other one doesn't know what to do or even think, because he or she is truly lost without the other half.

During courtship and falling in love, it is not uncommon for couples to become somewhat merged as they explore all the ways they are alike. It is healthy and normal, however, to let individual autonomy emerge as the couple discovers their differences in later phases of courtship. It is at this point that couples either break up—not wanting to "unmerge," and mistakenly thinking that differences mean there is something wrong with or incompatible in their relationship—or they unmerge and work to appreciate each other's unique qualities and how those qualities enhance the budding relationship. They desire individuality in their relationship in a way Merged couples do not.

Some couples evolve into a Merged relationship if they are together for a long time and fail to develop individual interests or receive support for individual growth.

Younger couples, too, can become merged—especially teenaged brides and grooms who wed before their individual personalities are fully formed. Chet and Sue came together at this early stage. Their story illustrates how the Merged Style does not support individuality and how change is challenging.

Chet and Sue first met in their ninth-grade science class as lab partners. Each describes their meeting as love at first sight. They were inseparable throughout high school. They signed up for the same classes and attended the same after-school activities. When Chet made the football team, Sue became a cheerleader. Because they spent the majority of their free time together, neither one of them developed close friendships outside their relationship. Sue loved Chet's sense of humor, and he can still make her laugh. He loves to be around her and thinks she is beautiful.

Chet developed skills as a carpenter while working at his father's construction company during summer breaks. Sue went to work at a local pharmacy. They married the summer after they graduated from high school, and in the next four years had two children. Sue continues to work part time. They are both loyal and valued workers at their respective jobs. Their life together has been fairly uneventful. They both follow the same daily routines and even go to the same resort for their yearly vacation. They spent ten years in this fashion. Then a change occurred.

The small construction firm at which Chet worked since graduating from high school expanded to several surrounding states. As lead carpenter, Chet is now required to oversee a number of these projects. He spends many weekdays at motels near the worksites and comes home on the weekends. As a result, Chet and Sue are both spending time on their own as they never had before in their relationship. Sue feels that she has nothing to do when Chet is away. She has made no significant friendships and has developed no personal interests. She says that she feels as though doing so would be disloyal to Chet. Sue found herself asking, "Is this all there is?" She is growing dissatisfied with what she calls "the same day over and over again," but she is unable to define what she would like to change. She feels that she is living for the weekends, when Chet is home.

Although Chet and Sue thought it was romantic to be so intertwined when they first got together—believing they are "two against the world"— Sue is finding it difficult to develop new interests while Chet is away during the week. Like Sue, who functions well at work and around her family, Chet is able to function separately from Sue on the job, but he doesn't enjoy his time with the guys on the site or even think to make friends. He harbors feelings that the other guys may not like him or want to socialize with him after work, so he turns down their invitations to go for burgers, beer, and pool when the workday is done. He's not used to socializing without Sue and is uncomfortable on his own. He relies on his weekend time with Sue to recharge his batteries, which is putting great stress on their marriage.

Like Chet and Sue, many Merged couples are limited to a narrow range of behaviors and interactions. They have developed few skills to identify their individual feelings, wants, and needs. When they are on their own, they are not able to define and verbalize their dissatisfaction and loneliness. When they step outside their merged bounds, they are often "lost." Chet feels lost away from Sue and cannot connect to his co-workers, so he focuses on work during the day and watches television in his motel room at night. Sue has only a limited ability to expand her activities and continues to feel unfulfilled on her own during the week. Chet clings to Sue when he is home on the weekends, and she wants more help with the children and to spend romantic time alone together. Neither of them has any idea how to change their pattern.

When they're alone, the individuals in a Merged couple feel vulnerable. They only feel whole and safe when they are together. If we imagine couples in the context of the larger world, such interdependence requires that neither of the Merged partners grow personally nor develop outside interests. They must rely on keeping the spark and continuing to interest each other, just as they are, with no surprises, changes, or uniqueness. Such limitations cause great strain, especially if one person desires more.

Decision making for the Merged couple occurs by unconsciously doing what the couple feels is typically expected of a husband or wife or partner without giving much thought to other options. Chet and Sue made most of their major decisions early in their relationship and seldom questioned them until their situation changed. In addition, without an awareness of individual needs and feelings, the Merged couple is not able to understand and share true intimacy, which requires the coming together of two whole, mature selves who are growing and changing, who support these processes in each other, and who are also developing new interests together over time.

## In the Merged Style

Decisions appear to be made early in the relationship and then stuck to indefinitely or until one person becomes dissatisfied. At that point, it is difficult for this couple to learn new patterns, because first, the partners must learn to be whole, individual adults, and then they must learn to be interdependent in healthy ways. Decisions for this couple are made unconsciously by adhering to what the couple feels is typically expected of people when they fall in love and marry. The couple appears to always agree, but the agreements are within a narrow range of what the partners think are acceptable. In the Merged relationship, the two people are fused, rather than separate individuals intimately connected through communication and interaction. They spend a lot of time together but do not know how to be apart. This merging is not developmentally healthy for either of them. It also limits the potential for developing a mature intimacy. Therefore, they may think they are emotionally connected, but they are not truly intimate by definition.

## The Roommate Style

The third model of relating applies not only to actual roommates and friends, but also to long-term couples. When applied to couples in a long-term romantic relationship, the Roommate Style typically describes two people of equal power and competence who share a home and other significant aspects of their lives. In addition to living together, they typically have sex, share some friends, and may even have a child. A major defining characteristic of the Roommate Style is that individuals in the couple make decisions unilaterally, without taking the partner into consideration; they may do this consciously or unconsciously. Some profess to value independence, but they do not balance it with interdependence that is necessary in any healthy, mature relationship.

For instance, a woman may come home one evening and tell her partner she's going out with her friends on Friday night (implying that he has to watch the kids, get a sitter, or fend for himself). A man might not feel it necessary to consult his partner when he chooses to quit or change his job. Perhaps they have separate finances, or it is assumed that the other partner will make financial adjustments as necessary.

Let's look at the relationship of Rahlah and Jeremy: They met through mutual friends and have been married for four years. Jeremy is fully engaged in his architectural career, and except for a serious college romance, had

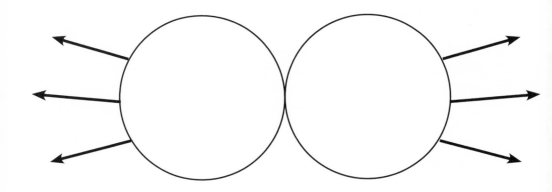

*In the Roommate Style of relationship, individuals are relatively equal in strength and power. They may share many things, but they make decisions unilaterally; connection happens randomly.*

not sought a long-term commitment until he met Rahlah. Like Jeremy, Rahlah is in her early thirties. She owns a small dot-com company through which she has been making and selling environmentally-friendly cleaning products for more than ten years. Jeremy was attracted to many of Rahlah's qualities, and he was especially impressed by her independence.

When Jeremy was offered a position with a prestigious firm on the East Coast, he was thrilled and accepted the offer without talking it over with his wife. Rahlah was delighted for him, and she was not in the least disturbed that her husband had not consulted her before making the decision to move several states away. Rahlah was confident that her business would do well "no matter where we live," and she enjoys that her husband is "as independent as I am." They have chosen to put off having children; Rahlah, however, thinks they should reconsider even having children at all due to her age. She is aware that having kids will require adjustments in their lifestyle, and this concerned her:

> I'm afraid we are both so independent—so focused on ourselves and our careers—that we won't know how to work together if we have kids. I'm afraid I'll end up taking care of the kids and the household even though I have a career, simply because we've never had to make decisions together

or put anyone else's needs before our own. I think we'd have to make a change in how we do things, but I'm not sure Jeremy sees the need for a change. He's doing just what he's always wanted to do, and he loves his job. Even though he really wants a family, I'm afraid he might not face just how much time kids require. He just thinks it will all work out. I'm concerned I'll have to pick up the slack and my needs will go on the back burner—not because he wants me to be overburdened or unhappy, but because it's what he's used to in our relationship. We've got it pretty good right now. I don't want to end up resenting him—or the kids.

Neither Rahlah nor Jeremy is dissatisfied with the amount of connection and intimacy they currently have because they are both so involved with their work lives. When they do come together, it is satisfying. Rahlah, however, is anticipating that if they have children she may desire more participation from Jeremy, as well as more connection and intimacy with him. The Roommate Style of relating may no longer be satisfying to her.

Like Jeremy and Rahlah, partners in the Roommate Style of relating come and go pretty much at will. This is done with the expectation that the other person, and maybe even the children, will make necessary adjustments without any discussion. Sometimes this works, and people are happy with the outcome; but when it doesn't work, at least one person will be left unhappy and, sometimes, unaware of what is wrong.

What distinguishes these relationships is the independent activity of each person. Each makes solo decisions, even when decisions affect both partners—and perhaps an entire family. Decision making is one-sided, even when the deciding partner has the best of intentions and feels that he or she is accommodating the partner's unspoken desires.

Another defining characteristic of the Roommate Style is that opportunities for emotional connection occur only randomly, because partners tend to function independently. There might be a steady connection at some times but only a sporadic connection at others. Partners cannot count on feeling emotionally connected to each other; and often a partner cannot count on the other person doing what he or she might choose to do for an activity, because each is used to making plans separately. Therefore, if they both wish to spend time together on Tuesday evening after work, the connection time is satisfying to both of them. Whether they are able to feel emotionally connected cannot be counted on, however—sometimes it may happen, and sometimes not.

While some couples consciously choose the Roommate Style, many don't actually set out to become Roommates. Those who consciously choose to act as Roommates tell me they value their independence. They seem to feel that relying on each other will take something away from their individuality. Therefore, they stridently talk about independent decision making. Frequently these couples become emotionally disconnected.

The couples that unconsciously fall into the Roommate Style of relating often tell me they simply think it is working for them. Sometimes it does when they are both choosing to be together and when they are both involved in other activities at the exact same time.

Modern couples with their busy lifestyles, careers, and family responsibilities often fall into this style by default rather than choice. Many of them have never really learned how to build and sustain a truly intimate partnership. Perhaps they saw their parents relating in this way, or the Roommate Style may have unconsciously developed as a way to avoid closeness—the result of previous disappointments and the inability to trust. Some of my clients point out that the Roommate Style can result from having to be strong and independent in their jobs and careers, which filter into the relationship.

Some couples have relative success in the Roommate Style when life is going fairly smoothly. I have also heard of couples being satisfied with this model when one or both have easygoing, non-goal-oriented personalities. Typically, this relaxed attitude is accompanied by knowledge that "my partner probably wouldn't change even if I asked him." Alternatively, as in any of the previous styles of relating, one or both individuals are conflict-avoidant, and they simply settle for being Roommates because they don't know what else to do to feel more satisfied. Because partners cannot always count on connecting with each other, the Roommate Style often leads to misunderstanding and dissatisfaction for one or both people.

As you've read Chapter 1 of *Romance Rehab* you've probably begun to identify some of the ways you relate that have led you to desire change. In the next chapter, you'll be introduced to another style of relating called Big Picture Partnering. This may be the style of relating you've been longing for.

## In the Roommate Style

Decision making is unilateral. Each person makes decisions individually, without necessarily consulting the other. The expectation is that one partner will adjust to the decisions made by the other. Opportunities for independence and individuality are high; interdependence is low. Emotional connections may happen frequently, intermittently, or very seldom, depending on each person's choices at any given time. While there may be two whole individuals in the Roommate relationship, this style results in limited opportunities for intimacy building, at best.

## Chapter 2

# The Benefits of Big Picture Partnering

In Chapter 1, we discussed Traditional, Merged, and Roommate relationship styles. The fourth way of relating is the Big Picture Partnering Style. While couples in the other three partnering styles usually experience difficulties and dissatisfaction, couples in Big Picture Partnering will learn

- how to listen to each other and make decisions together;

- new ways to connect and stay connected;

- how to balance individuality and mutuality or interdependence—so you develop the best in yourself and what is most satisfying in your partnership;

- how to create what you want together.

Couples in a Traditional, Merged, Roommate, or combination style relationship who want to change are completely capable of creating a Big Picture Partnership. In Part II of this book I will show you how. This chapter gives you an overview of the benefits of Big Picture Partnering; then you will build your partnership step-by-step as you learn this approach.

## Two People, One Journey

In the Big Picture Partnering Style, you mutually create three worlds, which are encompassed in a larger partnering universe.

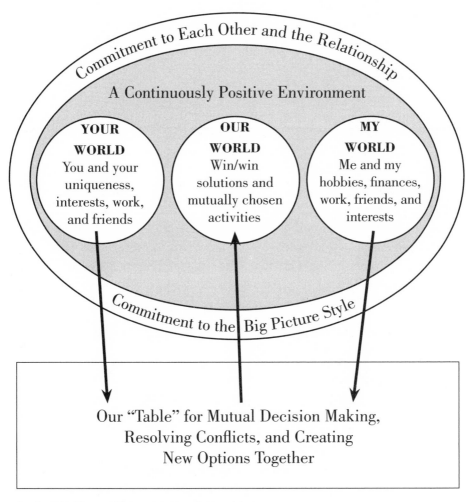

*In the Big Picture Universe your relationship is*

- *supported and strengthened by your commitments;*
- *nurtured by positive feelings, regular talking and listening, and essentials that build trust and connection;*
- *strengthened by your uniqueness—two lives, needs, desires, and dreams—which you bring to the relationship;*
- *solidified as you come together to create a mutually satisfying Our World; your issues and concerns, dreams, and desires go on the table for discussion; only win/ win solutions go into Our World.*

In this diagram, the circle on the left symbolizes Your World, which comprises all your individual uniqueness, friends, work, finances, activities, and so on; the circle on the right is Your Partner's World, which comprises all these aspects of your partner's life. Each of you has a high sense of individuality in this approach. The center circle—Our World—encompasses the mutually chosen and mutually created aspects of your life as a couple that only two unique human beings can build together.

The Our World circle represents the healthy interdependence you can have while retaining your individuality and some independence. The parts of your life that you share and enjoy together are in Our World. They are like the glue for your relationship. The Our World circle can include kids, house, mutual friends, finances, travel and vacation plans, hobbies or learning activities, religious or spiritual activities, exercising together, and so on. Our World contains elements that each couple agrees on together. Nothing goes into Our World unless it is a win/win, mutually satisfying decision.

You will notice in the diagram that there is a field surrounding the three worlds. This area is not a dead space. It is meant to represent the many positive behaviors and communications that keep your emotional connection alive. Outside of that field is a larger circle of commitments that protect your special relationship. Each element is indispensable in the Big Picture universe.

You will also notice in the diagram a table just outside the Our World circle. This symbolizes the Big Picture approach to communication and to reaching an agreement together. Rather than putting your concerns, disagreements, or differences between you, where they cause you to blame or become angry with and disconnected from each other, in Big Picture Partnering each partner brings thoughts, concerns, needs, wants, and desires to the table, where they are freely discussed as partnership concerns until the two of you arrive at a mutual decision about how you want to act.

Here's an example: Milo and Irina have been married thirteen years and have three children. Whenever Milo has a big decision to make about his work life, such as schedule or benefit changes that may affect his family, he brings it home and talks it over with Irina before committing to any major changes. He and Irina try to make all such major decisions together. "It may take us a little longer to talk everything over," he said, "but in the long run we are both happier. We are a family, and my job is, in many ways, 'our job.' Irina's happiness and the stability of our three kids is important to me. I value her opinion and really want her support in everything I do. So, we make these kinds of decisions together."

Unlike the previously described models of relating, in the Big Picture Partnering Style one world does not take away from another. Irina describes other aspects of their lives that she and Milo freely decide on—together, in the case of major decisions, such as finances, choice of schools for their children, or holiday plans with relatives, and separately, in the case of minor ones, such as calling the refrigerator repair technician or the youngest having a spontaneous sleepover with neighbor kids. They each realize that by choosing to be Big Picture Partners, no final decision is made if they are in disagreement about anything. The topic stays on the table for further discussion while they find other options that are mutually satisfying, win/win choices. That way, disagreements never stop or divide them. Irina said,

> I feel secure in knowing that we make all the major decisions together. We emigrated from Russia just after we were married, and I was pregnant. At the time we needed to be very connected—on everything—just to survive in this new country. We really learned how to work together. Over time, as we have become acclimated and at home here, we each have lots of separate activities— not only with the kids, but we are very social and have friends individually and couple friends together. Now that our six-year-old is in school, I have a part-time job, and this is my spending money separate from the family account. Milo takes his own allowance for his activities. I like to take pottery classes, and he is studying how to tutor other immigrants coming into the country. Along with our active kids, it makes for an exciting mix in our marriage!

In Big Picture Partnering, having two strong individual worlds, as Irina and Milo have, and an Our World together, is important. By learning and following the 10 Steps of Big Picture Partnering, summarized in the box on the next page, which you will learn during the coming chapters, all three worlds can coexist harmoniously. Using this approach, you will practice developing and balancing all three worlds in order to enjoy a richer and more rewarding relationship.

## The 10 Steps of Big Picture Partnering

Big Picture Partnering is an approach you will learn step-by-step in the coming chapters. Each step is like a building block so that eventually you will be using all 10 Steps in your rehab toolkit to keep your relationship strong and vibrant. These 10 Steps will become an integral part of your partnership, giving it a strong foundation. The tools you will learn are essential elements of the Big Picture Partnering approach. They are designed to help you support, nurture, protect, and express your relationship. While I encourage couples to incorporate other useful ideas for building and maintaining a wonderful partnership, if you do nothing else, follow these 10 Steps, and your relationship will become rock solid.

## 10 Steps to Rejuvenate Your Relationship

**Step 1:** Increase the Positive Between You

**Step 2:** Talk Regularly and Take Turns Listening

**Step 3:** Deepen Your Individuality to Strengthen Your Relationship

**Step 4:** Discover the Depth of Your Commitment

**Step 5:** Address Any Issue Together—Whether It's Yours, Mine, or Ours

**Step 6:** Understand How You Manage Conflict

**Step 7:** Put Your Issues on the Table so They Don't Come Between You

**Step 8:** Turn Problems into Mutual Goals and Work Toward Them Together

**Step 9:** Practice the Art of Heartfelt Listening

**Step 10:** Resolve Conflict and Create New Options Together

You and your partner will be guided in both individual and joint exercises to practice the 10 Steps in a building-block fashion. In each chapter, you will add a step one at a time and incorporate all ten by the end of the book. Some exercises will ask you to step back and look at the Big Picture of your relationship—what you value, desire, and envision. Others will require that you zoom in and focus on applying your Big Picture considerations and desires to the daily details of life—how you manage everything from household chores and schedules to finances, sexuality, and minor disagreements. The lessons in each chapter will build on the previous lessons until you gradually apply the tools of the Big Picture Partnering Style into your routines. As you incorporate these guidelines and tools, you will build together a rock-solid foundation for a satisfying relationship.

Most couples start with some combination of styles. As I mentioned earlier, the combination can be confusing if you unconsciously and randomly switch from one style to another. As you practice Big Picture Partnering, you will learn that it can include some elements that may look Traditional but are actually agreed upon as partners. For example, some couples adhere to the woman making the social plans and the man taking care of the lawn and the cars. If it is mutually agreed upon in their partnership, this is a Big Picture

## ✚ REHAB TOOLKIT
### What Is Our Style of Relating?

Which relationship style, or combination of styles, do you see you and your partner using in your relationship? Take one minute to do this individually in your notebook, then save your responses for further exercises later in this chapter.

Copy the following exercise into your notebook and fill in the blanks with the percentage of the time you feel that you and your partner spend in each style. (The four percentages should add up to 100 percent.)

| | |
|---|---|
| 1. Traditional Style | _____ % |
| 2. Merged Style | _____ % |
| 3. Roommate Style | _____ % |
| 4. Big Picture Partnering Style | _____ % |
| Total | =100% |

Reflect on your assessment of your relationship. Why did you choose each of these styles? Then think about how you would like your relationship to be. In the exercises at the end of this chapter you will share your assessment and your thoughts with your partner.

---

Partnering Style. Another example would be areas of great independence approved by both partners. You don't have to revert to being Roommates to achieve some independence. You simply need to learn to work toward what satisfies you individually and together—and arrive at the win/win solutions together.

## Making Decisions Together

When you choose the Big Picture Style, the way in which you and your partner make decisions is quite different from those of the other three styles. In the Big Picture, Our World decisions—those that involve both people—are made together. Your World and My World decisions are made individually but are supported by each partner.

In Big Picture Partnering, any issue can be brought to the table for discussion; however, nothing goes into the Our World circle until it is fully agreed upon by both individuals. Big Picture decision making is not necessarily about compromise. Neither is it about neglecting your own needs in order to attend to those of your partner. Rather, it challenges both partners to become imaginative and to recognize or invent new options together. This approach helps you master the fine art of blending each of your needs into something totally new and unique—an Our World that satisfies both of you.

One-time decisions—what to have for dinner, which movie to go to, or whether to stay home on Friday night—are easy. However, sometimes Big Picture Partnering means that couples will discuss and mull things over for a number of weeks. For instance, shortly after Marybeth and Ron were married, they began to pursue the topic of buying a house. It was a loaded topic because Marybeth wanted to live in the city, and Ron had always wanted a home on a lake. At the time, they found it hard to imagine how this situation might be resolved to the satisfaction of both, and they wanted to make sure neither of them settled or simply "gave in," knowing they'd be dealing with big resentments later.

## Decision Making Is a Big Deal

No matter how big or small your issues may seem, making decisions together is critical. Decisions may range from where to buy a house or how to divvy up household chores and childcare, all the way to healing from an affair or resolving a betrayal such as loss of financial stability or a job due to one partner's gambling or drinking. It's not the magnitude of the decision that is the tipping factor; it's how you make decisions. If one of you simply gives in, or settles, or compromises too much or too often, chances are resentments will arise sooner or later and undermine your relationship.

Agreeing to practice their partnering skills, Marybeth and Ron spent much time talking, looking, researching, and investigating their alternating openness and resistance to each other's desire. They took turns looking by lakes and in the city. Then they found a little dream home in an unexpected place—halfway between country and city.

The Big Picture Partnering skills—the 10 Steps—helped them put a new home into their Our World circle within eight months. They have had no regrets or resentments. Not long ago, Marybeth called,

> I am still surprised at how Ron and I were able to come together on a decision when we initially appeared to be so far apart in what we wanted. Our choice of a little house near one of the inner suburban lakes has pleased both of us.

Since purchasing the home nine years ago, Marybeth and Ron have partnered on many other decisions. They have remodeled and expanded their house and landscaped the yard; Ron moved his offices out of the house; and they are raising three boys and a family dog in it since they made their Our World decision.

## Connecting—and Staying Connected—in a New Way

How does Big Picture Partnering allow for a new kind of connection? The Big Picture Style does this by enhancing and drawing on each other's individuality—a primary requirement for true connection and intimacy. Big Picture relationships nurture emotional connection and provide many consistent opportunities for intimacy.

As you use the Big Picture approach, you will clearly experience the many and consistent opportunities for communication and connection that are built into partnering. At first you will be guided to communicate in small increments and to apply these communications to important daily basics. Gradually you will expand these skills as you apply them to deeper issues that may have been more difficult to resolve in your past. Then you will go on to apply your new communication skills to creating your future dreams together.

Communicating and interacting, in and of themselves, do not ensure that you will feel emotionally, mentally, or spiritually connected all the time. That is unrealistic. Take the example of Pete and Barb. Pete's role model was his dad, a verbally abusive alcoholic. While Pete was neither abusive nor alcoholic, under stress, such as when Barb thought they needed to spend money on the children's winter boots and finances were tight—not knowing another way— Pete reverted to the hostile refusal to discuss things he'd seen his dad use while growing up. At first, Barb tried to reason with him, but over time, she became more and more timid. Their relationship deteriorated. It didn't matter how big or small the issue or topic, they could not talk or connect on almost anything. In desperation, they turned to Big Picture Partnering and learned the 10 Steps. It didn't always feel good or easy to talk—and they didn't regenerate their longed-for, in-love feelings for many months as they talked through even the mundane things they had been unable to previously discuss. However, gradually a new sense of closeness developed as they consistently applied the tools you too will learn in this book.

Big Picture Partnering will help you create more opportunities for meaningful emotional connection, which is the stepping stone to intimacy. Using this approach, you will learn to connect frequently and consistently about everyday details as well as about your future Big Picture.

## Balancing Individuality and Mutuality

Big Picture Partners bring to their relationships two distinct and unique individual selves who consciously choose to be connected. They desire to support each other's strong sense of individuality while also promoting the mutual decisions of the Our World circle they create.

Some couples find this easy to do in the beginning of a relationship, but over time—especially when children or demanding work responsibilities are introduced—remembering to take some time for each of your personal interests and for each other can be challenging. What's important is to value each other's needs as much as you value your partnership and your children's needs. Then you aim for the best balance possible, which may vary from week to week as you try to squeeze in that workout, or spend time individually with your friends. Discounting or overlooking these needs for too long can lead to resentment. Children also do better when parents are caring for their own and each other's needs while also providing positive parenting.

When couples support and work to balance both individual and couple needs, the resulting relationship becomes a mutual creation made of the inspiration, imagination, personal histories, experiences, gifts, and resources of the two partners.

## Learning to Be Creative and Find New Options Together

Learning to come up with new options or solutions to your needs and problems is a skill you will want to learn through the 10 Steps in this book. Doing this together will make you feel good about yourselves and each other. The new options you invent together can be applied to everyday problems you face, such as who's going to do the meal planning, grocery shopping, and daily cooking when both of you work full time. Creative solutions are definitely required if this is your second marriage and you are trying to meld two households and one or two sets of kids, exes, and in-laws. Coming up with new options is also necessary as children get older and are able to participate in household chores or require more juggling of schedules as you take them to games or extracurricular activities.

As you learn to problem solve together and apply your creative options to everyday issues, these wrinkles will begin to smooth out. Once this happens, Big Picture Partners discover they then have more time to develop their Big Picture dreams together—no matter what your age or stage in relating.

Let me tell you about Harvey and Lenore. In their early fifties, each was on a second marriage. They had been together for seven years when I met them. "We are at a wonderful time of our lives and want to do something totally different," Harvey explained. "We just don't know what that is. All we know is we want to live in a warmer climate as we get older, and we want to do something more fun!" Lenore especially wanted to live in a smaller and more eco-friendly community. Neither of them was sure how to make these parts of their dream into a whole. "We'll probably make a change in five or six years," Harvey told me, not knowing the power of the Big Picture.

Harvey had been a successful corporate executive for many years, and he had a love of mountain climbing, which he seldom had time to do. He wanted to try something entrepreneurial and thought one avenue might be to offer training and consulting to companies in how to go through difficult changes. Or maybe he could write. Or . . . he really wasn't sure. Lenore worked as an office manager for a local arts organization and wanted to remain in the arts. She also wanted to explore her writing talent.

As they had discussions about their values and dreams, Harvey and Lenore eagerly began using the 10 Steps. They started to experiment with different job ideas and traveled to explore different parts of the country where they might live. After five months, they arrived at a totally unexpected plan, all due to their brainstorming, experimenting, and exploring. Here's how Harvey explained the process:

> We thought we would explore the temperate parts of the West Coast and ended up spending the last four weeks in Bend, Oregon. We met the nicest people, it's beautiful, and I've decided it's the perfect place to start a mountain-climbing and hiking business for anyone—maybe even corporate execs—with treks to Mt. Hood and the surrounding area.

Harvey was jazzed. It was entrepreneurial and different from his corporate job, yet it included knowledge of what execs might need. He had met some folks doing similar things in Bend, and they had invited him to explore building this aspect of their sporting company. Lenore had fallen in love with the high-desert climate and made friends with people in a local community organization that worked to protect the environment. She was enthusiastic about the area and her new job prospect:

> They need someone to help them organize and write for them. I'm good at both, and it would be about twenty-five hours a week so I could also work on my novel.

Within nine months, Harvey and Lenore were excitedly closing on the sale of their home in Minneapolis and moving to Oregon. They still write or call once in a while. In our last conversation, Lenore told me,

> I can't tell you how delighted we continue to be with the changes we made eleven years ago. To think that we could still be stuck in our old rut—but you got us working together and the changes happened so quickly. We are still both surprised.

## Daily Details and Big Picture Dreams

Why is it that we rarely manage to resolve with our partner those constant arguments about the little things in life? We spend so much energy hassling over whose turn it is to wash the dishes, why the kids aren't finishing their breakfast, or which set of in-laws to invite for the holidays.

Big Picture Partnering will provide you with a set of tools to apply solutions to daily problems. For each couple, the list of issues that cause frequent arguments will be different, but you'll do an inventory so you can pinpoint the ones that nag you the most. You'll cover everything from finances and chores to parenting, in-laws, friendships, and vacations.

You will be guided toward creative problem solving with your partner, so the two of you don't have to spend all of your energy on the same day-to-day problems. Former problem areas will become comfortable, agreed upon routines. As a result, your creative energies will be freed up for your Big Picture dreams and visions or for simply more fun and play.

## Your Big Picture Adventure

As you begin this adventure together, think about where you've been and where you might be headed. What has characterized your relationship to this point in your lives, and how would you like it to look a year from now?

Reflect on your assessment of styles of relating. Most people start out with a combination of styles and work toward becoming Big Picture Partners all the time. Partnering requires a lot of consciousness and a bit of effort, but the short- and long-term benefits are many.

In the coming chapters, I will walk you through all 10 Steps of Big Picture Partnering so you can learn to communicate, interact, and create the outcomes the two of you most desire. This process will sometimes lead—or even force—you to come up with entirely new and unexpected options. As you learn to partner, not only will you find yourselves discovering mutually agreeable solutions to previously unresolved problems, but also you'll enjoy more fun and spontaneity. As you apply the 10 Steps of Big Picture Partnering to such conflicts, you'll discover, to your delight, that the two of you have grown closer—and happier—in the process.

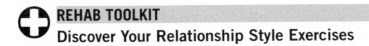

## REHAB TOOLKIT
## Discover Your Relationship Style Exercises

### The Styles of Relating on Your Family Tree

In the following exercises you will have the opportunity to reflect on the relationship influences you experienced growing up, as well as those in your extended-family history.

Each of you should individually make a sketch of your personal family tree. Begin with the branches closest to you, then your parents, grandparents, and great-grandparents. Don't forget to include members of blended families, especially step-parents.

Now look at your family tree. Identify which of the four styles of relating each of these couples modeled. (Some information may come from your direct experiences; some, from stories you've heard about these relatives.)

How do you think you were influenced or affected—positively and negatively—by these role models? When you think about the style of relating you would like to develop, how does your family tree influence your current choices? Write about your reflections in your notebook. You will share with your partner shortly.

### Bringing Your Relationship Experience Together

At this point, come together to share and compare your responses to the individual exercises you completed within this chapter. As you share your responses to these exercises, simply listen to each other.

First share with each other your lists of what is happening when things are going well between you and when things are not going well. Simply note where you are similar.

Then place your family trees next to each other. Take turns describing the influences that come from your respective family histories. Again, listen quietly and carefully as you each share your family patterns and how they had an impact on you when relating both positively and negatively.

Then take out your assessment of styles of your current relationship. Tell each other which style or combination of styles you think typifies your relationship right now. Does your relationship most resemble the Traditional, Merged, Roommate, or

Big Picture Partnering Style, or some combination of these four? Tell your partner why you chose each style in your assessment. Listen to each other's experience and talk about how your relationship has evolved over time. What were the various turning points, such as having a child, a promotion at work that led to longer hours, a family illness, a friend's divorce, and so on, when the underlying style changed? Can you identify together what might have caused the change?

Take turns talking and listening to how you scored the various styles and what is satisfying or dissatisfying. Then listen especially to each other's dreams about whether you are satisfied with the style of relating that characterizes your relationship today.

Look at both your relationship as a whole, then various aspects of it (communication, conflict resolution, shared interests, sex life, household management, etc.). Take turns talking about how you would like your relationship style to change. Write your responses and what you learned in your notebook. Save what you've written to help you work toward becoming more loving and intimate partners in the coming weeks as you incorporate the 10 Steps of Big Picture Partnering.

# The 10 Steps to Your Best Relationship

In Part I of *Romance Rehab* you were encouraged to think about your "big picture" as you became acquainted with four different styles of relating. You read about the Traditional, Merged, and Roommate styles that couples often adopt either by default or as a result of prior role modeling. You learned how these three styles can lead to discontent and dissatisfaction. Then you were introduced to the Big Picture Partnering Style and its benefits. Finally, exercises guided you to evaluate your current relationship style and to reflect on how you'd really like it to be.

I hope your horizons are expanding with these new ways of thinking about yourselves as a couple. Maybe you gained some understanding of potential reasons you may be stuck or in a rut. I also suspect you feel a glimmer of hope that things can change. At the same time, you are probably feeling a bit skeptical about how to make these changes, and rightly so. Now you need the tools to work in sync as partners and resolve whatever problems you face to create the future you want together.

Part II of *Romance Rehab* will teach you the 10 Steps to create the change you most desire. The steps are the basic tools to practice together and use forever. They are taught as building blocks you add one at a time to your repertoire. They will help you resolve problems, keep your relationship rock-solid, and show you how to become inventive together as you seek win/win solutions.

## Chapter 3

# STEP 1:

## Increase the Positive Between You

You want to rehabilitate or rejuvenate your relationship. You've just been introduced to the Big Picture Partnering Style. Theoretically, it may sound wonderful—just what you desire—but easier said than done. "Sounds good, but how do we get from 'here' to 'there'?" you ask. You will do it by taking it one step at a time. The next step is to remember the good things that brought you together in the first place.

This week you will learn about **Big Picture Step 1: Increase the Positive Between You.** You will be guided to remember the positive interactions that brought you together and to reflect on why you may have discontinued your courtship. If you have been fighting, you will be asked to stop fighting for now while you learn a more effective way of resolving your problems. To rehab or reinvigorate your relationship, focusing on the positive will prepare you for the partnering tools and new solutions you will develop as you work through all 10 Steps in this book. As you become consciously aware of your positive impact on the relationship, you will feel empowered to create a safe and nurturing environment even when there are issues to discuss or outside stresses. By emphasizing the positive, you will naturally feel good about yourself, your partner, and your relationship—and you'll have more energy to face any issues together.

## How the 5-to-1 Ratio Affects Every Couple

One of the ways couples have been studied over the last thirty years is in a laboratory setting, sometimes with observers taking notes behind a one-way mirror; at other times the couples are videotaped. In either approach, specific behaviors are then methodically counted and analyzed for their impact on the overall quality of the relationship. Ultimately, these studies search for ways to help couples maximize the positives that help relationships endure.

In the 1990s, such meticulous observation from a number of well-known research labs around the country yielded a wealth of data to back up the therapy and coaching methods many professionals were successfully, and sometimes not so successfully, using.

One of the most consistently published and publicized professionals bringing forth this valuable data is John M. Gottman, PhD, the cofounder and codirector of the Seattle Marital and Family Institute and professor of psychology at the University of Washington. He has studied thousands of couples and is able to predict with 87 percent accuracy which marriages are headed for divorce within three years. He is also 81 percent accurate in predicting which marriages will survive after seven to nine years.

As summarized in his book, *Why Marriages Succeed or Fail*, one of the major factors in the endurance of relationships is the number of times certain behaviors are exhibited. High on Gottman's list of couple-success factors are positive feelings and interactions that nourish a relationship and fortify it in times of outside stress.

According to Gottman,

> The magic ratio is 5-to-1. In other words, as long as there is five times as much positive feeling and interaction between husband and wife as there is negative, we found the marriage was likely to be stable. It was based on this ratio that we were able to predict whether couples were likely to divorce: In very unhappy couples, there tended to be more negative than positive interaction.

He goes on to identify negative emotions as, among others, anger, contempt, criticism, and defensiveness. The positive side of the equation is defined as showing interest, affection, appreciation, concern, and empathy; being accepting; joking around when it is fun for both; and sharing joy. In Gottman's research, it doesn't matter how much arguing there is overall; what matters is that the positive interactions far outshine any negativity.

## How the 5-to-1 Ratio Makes Your Partnership Rock-Solid

We all know that when we are in the honeymoon phase of a new relationship, we engage in our best behavior. We are "tuned in" and attentive to the other person as a new friendship or love relationship develops. Positive interactions are typically very high. While we are not consciously aware of keeping the negatives low, we unconsciously try to show our best side. This ratio of high positives in the beginning of any relationship is what keeps us coming back for more.

Jaime and Jonathan began their relationship with just such a scenario, but by the time they came to see me, they described an erratic emotional connection. They had dated for two years before they married. Their first daughter was born within a year, and the second arrived within two years. Now, ten years later, Jaime runs her own research and consulting business from home. Jonathan is a middle manager at a local firm. They both agree that their relationship has been a committed one, but it has run hot and cold ever since they were engaged. They talked about stretches of time when relating was smooth. Jaime volunteered,

> During those times we get along, the house and schedules run well. We even have a lot of playfulness together, and with the kids. Of course, there's more sex!

Jonathan added,

> And then we seem to hit a wall. I don't know why it keeps happening. One of us gets hurt or angry, or an old issue resurfaces. Then the cold war starts. Of course I always think she starts it, but when it's over I know that isn't true. Sometimes it goes on for a few days, and sometimes it can stretch into two weeks. We each want the other person to apologize or warm up, but we are both pretty stubborn people. I don't even know what makes us get over it, but eventually we do. Maybe the problems go underground and we just go on. We really like each other, so eventually we give up the silent fight. I just wish we'd get over it sooner, and maybe get to the bottom of what is bugging us.

Jaime for the most part shared Jonathan's concerns:

> We'd both like to figure this out. It's tiring, and I get lonelier and lonelier every time it happens. I think this is because life is pretty demanding as the

girls get older and our schedules include all of their activities as well as our own. The kids notice it too. I'd just like this to smooth out. Besides, he's my buddy—except when I'm upset and shut down or he's aloof and ignoring me.

When I asked Jaime and Jonathan to talk about what drew them together ten years ago, they took turns quickly coming up with substantial lists of things they liked about each other and enjoyed doing together. Jaime cited Jonathan's little courtesies, like opening doors for her or bringing her flowers, and she loved his sense of humor: "Gosh, could he make me laugh! He still does, when we are getting along."

Jonathan recalled how upbeat she was and how she made him feel special: "She was interested in knowing everything about me; I loved the way she looked at me."

"And what about intelligence, depth, and attraction?" I prompted, seeing that they were both good-looking, fit, and smart. Jaime laughed,

> Oh that! I take it for granted that he's smart. I couldn't be with a man unless he was a thinker. Jonathan is thoughtful, bright, and we share the same values. I've never stopped thinking he is a hunk!

Jonathan interjected,

> Jaime is downright beautiful, even in her jeans or sweats. I've always thought so. I guess I just don't tell her often enough anymore.

This statement became a turning point. Although a bit hesitant at first, Jaime and Jonathan began to link their earlier ability to show appreciation and to please each other with the drought in their current relationship. They realized how little they appreciated or tried to overtly please each other regularly anymore.

In the beginning, Jaime and Jonathan's positive interactions far outweighed their negative interactions—just as John Gottman advises. So they knew how to be more positive with each other; they just needed to put into practice what they already knew. Their assignment was to achieve five or more positive interactions for every negative one. Doing so empowered them to quickly improve their relationship and put it back on a positive track in a way that took very little effort. Consistently feeling better about themselves and each other then helped them create a stronger, and even happier, partnership in the months to come as they learned the Big Picture approach.

Just like Jaime and Jonathan, we know that during the honeymoon phase couples put their best foot forward. We also know that the longer we interact with another person, the closer we become and the more we reveal aspects of our personality, attitudes, and behavior. As the honeymoon wanes, we gradually feel more comfortable, letting down our guard. At the same time, the longer we know someone—especially the one we are closest to—the more often we take each other for granted. It is not unusual for people to treat colleagues and acquaintances with more kindness and respect than those they live with and love the most. It is not uncommon to see friends or workmates receiving the best time and the most high-quality interactions, while mate and family members receive the leftovers.

## REHAB TOOLKIT
## Household Agreements Consistently Keep Your Positives High

In any household certain behaviors should be expected; you should be able to count on them. Examples may include

- frequent "I love you's";

- kisses and hugs hello and good-bye (and good morning and good night);

- saying "please" and "thank-you";

- never going to bed angry;

- never discussing difficult topics before 8:00 a.m. or after 8:00 p.m.;

- requesting attention instead of demanding or expecting it if your partner or family member is busy;

- turning off the cell phone or stepping away from the computer or television when your spouse or family member speaks to you;

- asking if it is okay to interrupt a task you are in the middle of.

I recommend couples come together and make a list of "Household Agreements" that everyone in the family abides by at all times. Such expectations will automatically keep your positive interactions high. Make a list together. If you have children, invite them to add their ideas to your list. That way they know that the list of expected behaviors applies to everyone in the family—including you!

## When the Negative Outweighs the Positive

The following are excerpts from first sessions with couples whose lack of positive interactions emphasized the negative:

Sarah and Will had been married for nine years, but Sarah found herself increasingly unhappy with their Traditional Style relationship:

> Will frequently comes home late from work, and I'm disappointed when he misses a great dinner I've prepared. Sometimes he even forgets the kids' baseball games. They are always so proud when he shows up, but I can tell they try not to get their hopes up, because we just can't count on him these days. He puts work first.

Ramona's eleven-year marriage to Carl was a Merged/Roommate Style before they learned Big Picture Partnering. Here, she noted how the relationship shifted from high positives to a preponderance of negatives:

> Carl was such a gentleman when we first knew each other. He'd not only open doors and spend time with me, but he actually talked to me every day—like he really wanted to and enjoyed it. Now all he does is joke about my weight or talk sarcastically about my work. He gets lost in the television or some household chore when I want more time for talk and affection.

Conversely, Paul, married thirteen years to Lynette, assessed their relationship style as strictly Roommate:

> Lynette cleans house every night, long after I've gone to bed. I feel like she puts the chores before me—and I feel ignored. She always says she'll come to bed early, and I know she feels guilty. But she doesn't change her behavior.

Other couples note that while their partners are still playful and funny with friends and colleagues, that same bond that once connected them as a couple has vanished, replaced by a willful distance. Maybe you recognize such diminishing positives in your relationship.

As these couples demonstrate, when negative interactions in a relationship outweigh positive, partners usually feel unappreciated. At first some partners may not notice or react to a lack of positive interaction—or to a lack of any interaction at all. Over time, however, a lack of positives brings out feelings of sadness, rejection, withdrawal, and eventually depression or anger or both.

Typically this behavior begins a negative pattern as the partner who is hurting tries to reach out for connection, sometimes gently at first, but eventually turns to other negative interactions such as angry outbursts or demands for attention. The partner who has withdrawn affection and appreciation may have angry, defensive outbursts in return or may shut down even further. Either way, such negative interactions quickly snowball and spiral downward. They become a repetitive cycle of withdrawal or a vicious cycle of shaming, blaming, criticizing, and anger toward each other.

## You Hold the Key

No couple wants to be caught in such a cycle of negativity—and you can get yourself out of this predicament. By consistently creating and maintaining positive feelings, and then building on those good feelings, the Big Picture Partnering approach will help you avoid or break out of such a negative pattern. When we stop nourishing our relationship—when we put our love relationship last on the list of priorities—love, and the ultimate success of our most important relationship, is at stake.

---

TIP: In keeping with the research on successful relationships, Big Picture partners maintain a 5-to-1 ratio or better of positive-to-negative interactions. This is their insurance policy, the emotional savings account that sustains them during times of stress. It is their consistent investment that reflects the high priority they give their partnership.

---

In Big Picture Partnering, if you have one argument, or one tense or stressful interaction within a day or a week, you need at least five positive interactions within that same period of time. If you have four difficult, heated, or argumentative interactions, you need twenty positive interactions.

A positive interaction may be a hug, a pat on the back, making a nice dinner, doing a favor, making love, saying something nice to your partner, being willing to resolve a difficult situation by staying "present" in a conversation, and so on. Positive interactions that outweigh negative ones are defined as those considered positive in the eyes of you and your partner. Going to a B&B for the weekend, gifts, or flowers do count as positives in this equation. In most couples I see, however, the positives that really matter are the small acts of kindness, thoughtfulness, and generosity—going out of your way for an errand,

## ✚ REHAB TOOLKIT
## Our Positive/Negative Ratio

Reflect on the many interactions between you and your partner in the past six weeks. Answer the following questions in your notebook. Complete this exercise on your own. Later this week you will be asked to come together to share your responses.

Think about the number of positive interactions you and your partner have had in the course of a week. (Just use your best estimate.)

- In the past six weeks, my partner and I have had approximately _____ (number) positive interactions each week.

Think about the number of negative interactions you and your partner have experienced in the past six weeks. (Again, if needed, just use your best estimate.)

- In the past six weeks, my partner and I have had approximately _____ (number) negative interactions each week.

Now compare these two numbers and determine a ratio between the two:

- My estimate of our Positive-to-Negative Ratio is _____positive / _____negative.

On your own, reflect and write about this ratio and how it compares to Gottman's research. According to Gottman's findings (five or more positives are needed for every one negative interaction), what does your score indicate to you? A "High Positives" ratio is desirable and, of course, the ratio of positives to negatives can always be increased! Do you have an abundance or a deficit? If you are in deficit, reflect on when this started and how you contribute to the negativity between you.

---

coming home early from the office, making that extra phone call home to check in, taking time for sex even if the house needs cleaning.

## Please Your Partner and Increase Your Pleasure Together

Sometimes couples are in great upheaval or pain. They may have significant issues that they are attempting to resolve. They may mistakenly imagine that it helps to discuss these issues repeatedly and constantly. They want to resolve the problem but it is not working. They argue a topic over and over until they can no longer do anything pleasant together. In this situation, a couple's positive-to-negative ratio is totally unbalanced, and their relationship nourishment is empty, inhibiting resolution.

# ✚ REHAB TOOLKIT
## Pleasing My Partner

Stop a minute to reflect on your relationship. At this point, do not share your thoughts with your partner; simply write in a notebook. Do not analyze, comment, or judge your reflections. There are no right or wrong answers. You will be asked to share your thoughts with each other in the exercises at the end of this chapter.

- Make a list of four ways you currently please your partner.

- Make a list of four things your partner does that you appreciate.

- What are two or three things your partner would like you to do that you know would be appreciated if you did them (because he has stated so, or she has made the request), or if you did them more often?

- Privately reflect on your reasons for not doing the things your partner would appreciate and ask yourself, might I be willing to consider these requests as things I might do to increase the positives between us?

---

If you are in this negative pattern it may feel difficult to refocus yourselves as a couple, to reverse the positive-to-negative ratio. You may be afraid the issues will never be addressed. Be reassured that the issues will be attended to in time. First, however, you must nourish your relationship by implementing Step 1, expanding the positive interactions between you. If you are willing to lay down your arms, put your fights on hold, and increase the positive interactions, you will calm your relationship and start to feel more connected again. Then you can learn more tools to revisit what has been difficult between you in a more effective and productive—and successful—way.

Your relationship may be stronger and less stressful than the couples I have just described. Even if that's the case, however, it is crucial to continue to nourish your relationship. Without positive feelings, we have less desire to give or to work on problematic areas. We succumb to waiting for the other person to change first. A nourishing environment of positive feelings gives us the energy to deal with situations that arise. What appeared to be a big issue or problem suddenly seems doable, smaller, less threatening. We feel more spontaneous and playful. Our relationship feels sweeter, juicier.

We all know what to do to please our partners. Each of us has a wealth of experience. Once the honeymoon is over, however, some people act as if they forgot, don't know, or don't remember what makes their partner happy, even though they have observed happy, excited, or pleased responses at other times during their relationship. When I challenge couples on this point, asking them to make lists or say out loud the things that please their partner, they come up with at least four or five items they are sure of. This is a start. If they have forgotten what pleases their partner, I encourage them to ask.

When you go out of your way to do something that pleases your partner, you both can reap the benefits.

In Big Picture Partnering, partners are encouraged to have a healthy repertoire of "positives" they can carry out and interchange regularly, so that positive interactions become like breathing—natural, regular, easy, and always nourishing the two people involved. The exercises at the end of the chapter will help you increase your positive interactions to five or more for every negative you encounter.

## Stop Fighting for Now

As you work to rejuvenate your most important love relationship, I am going to ask those of you who fight about issues that remain unresolved to stop fighting for now. If your fights are frequently unresolved, it means you do not yet have the tools to be successful working together. As you work toward becoming Big Picture Partners, you will practice the 10 Steps in this book. These are steps you can use for a lifetime—to calm your relationship, increase the positive feelings between you, and then communicate in new ways about previously unresolved differences.

Once you stop fighting and feel more positive, you will learn the tools to tackle your unresolved problems and issues. These 10 Steps will help you re-approach any issues that have been problematic. Built into the 10 Steps are new and safe ways to talk about difficult topics. As you proceed, some differences or disagreements may even seem less problematic. For the time being, bite your tongues, write in your notebook, go for a walk, and, most important, make a pact with each other to learn how to communicate better— to communicate for resolution and with imagination as you go through this process.

If you have been fighting, you will be directed to sign a pact to stop fighting for now in the exercises that follow. You will individually make a list of the topics that you are fighting about, unresolved issues, and anything you want to be different between you. You will not share this list. Instead, you will put this list and these fights aside for a few weeks while you learn and practice new ways of connecting. We will revisit these lists later in this program as you turn your problems into goals and action plans so they can be mutually resolved.

## Warning

When you stop fighting you may feel sad or hurt for a while. Some people even become depressed. This is because anger and rage typically cover up your underlying helplessness, hopelessness, discouragement, and sorrow. Allow yourself to go into these quieter feelings if you have been experiencing a lot of anger. You might choose to write in your notebook about what you are unhappy about. Go to the deepest level. I suspect you had great hopes and dreams that may have been dashed. You may be experiencing sadness at your own behavior, and great disappointment in your partner. You may feel like your partner is not there for you. Are you there for your partner?

If you let yourself sink into your sadness and start to feel depressed, remember that depression is a state of being rather than an emotion. Sadness is an emotion that can ebb and flow from one minute or one hour to the next. Do not hang onto any feelings you may have and don't be discouraged if you do feel a little depressed. Be sure to eat healthy foods, get enough sleep, exercise often, and spend time in the sunshine to help avoid depression.

If you are not too disconnected from your partner, staying in your sadness instead of your anger can allow you to gently and tenderly connect. You can do this simply by sharing meals, holding hands while going for a walk, and maybe cuddling at bedtime without being sexual. This can help you feel some connection, even without words.

# REHAB TOOLKIT
## Step 1 Exercises

### Awareness of Positives and Feeling Loved

Now that you have read and reflected on the importance of positive feelings and interactions in your relationship, write in your notebook and refer to the Our Positive-to-Negative Ratio exercise on page 39. Reflect on your individual assessment of this ratio once again. Each of you should ask yourself, "What is the positive-to-negative ratio in my partnership now? What do I do to make it higher or lower? If I notice I am withholding something—affection, time, attention, sex, talk, play, or anything else I know would please my partner—why is that? What are my concerns or motivations for not keeping the good feelings flowing? Am I waiting for my partner to go first? What attitudes and behaviors do I need to change to see or do this differently? What could I do (no matter what my partner is doing) to enhance this base of good feeling within my partnership?"

Be sure to include in your self-assessment your responses from the Pleasing My Partner exercise on page 40.

Refine your awareness of what pleases you and your partner as you each continue to write in your notebook. Write about those actions your partner already does that you appreciate, that make you feel cared for or loved.

Then contemplate what you think satisfies your partner. What makes each of us feel loved is unique; often, we assume that what makes us feel loved also makes our partner feel loved. Ask yourself, "Am I willing to learn from my partner how to express my love in the way he or she most appreciates?"

### Expanding Your Loving

Another time, take turns sharing your lists of things your partner does that you appreciate and what you do out of caring, from the Pleasing My Partner exercise on page 40. Listen carefully to what makes each of you feel loved by the other.

Next, share what your partner has requested and have your partner clarify for you why these things would feel especially good. Be sure to listen carefully and non-defensively if the requests have been difficult in the past. Remember, this is not a demand. The intention is to learn what pleases your partner. Sometimes this is different from what pleases you.

Then create and give each other another list of additional pleasing actions. Be specific. For example, you might say, "I really enjoy when you arrange for the babysitter and pick the movie on our night out." Or, "When you call me during the day just to say hello, I feel very cared for." Or, "I love it when you tease me with your toes under the tablecloth when we're eating in a nice restaurant."

Invest in your relationship. Expand the positive—your love repertoire—together.

---

✚ **REHAB TOOLKIT**
## Signing Our "Do Not Fight" Pact

Whether you have been fighting or not, copy and sign this agreement with each other.

We, _____ and _____, agree to discontinue fighting about hot topics, big problems, and unresolved issues while we practice becoming more intimate Big Picture Partners. We do this knowing we will have ample opportunity to discuss these issues—with improved communication ability—as we integrate all 10 Steps in the coming weeks.

Signed _____     Signed _____
Date _____     Date _____

NOTE: If your partner is not ready to participate or to sign the agreement and you are, sign it and make the commitment anyway. You can begin to make the changes on your own, and they will have an impact on how you feel about yourself and pave the way for changes in your relationship, even if you have to go it alone.

### Putting Our Disagreements Aside—For Now

Individually, make a list of the topics you are fighting about, issues that are unresolved, anything that you want to be different between you. You will not share this list right now. Instead, you will put this list and these fights aside for a few weeks while you learn and practice new ways of connecting. Put the list in an envelope or at the back of your notebook, but save it. You will revisit this list a number of times later in this program as you turn your problems into goals and action plans so they can become mutually resolved, win/win solutions that satisfy both of you.

**Chapter 4**

# STEP 2:
## Talk Regularly and Take Turns Listening

While you continue to practice Step 1, nourishing your relationship by increasing positive interactions between you, in this chapter you will learn about **Big Picture Step 2: Talk Regularly and Take Turns Listening**. Step 2 places an emphasis on creating a consistent thread of meaningful communication that you can sustain at all times—especially during busy and stressful times.

I am continually surprised by the variation in the amount of time couples spend talking to each other. Some couples barely see each other during the week. Taking an extra five minutes a day to talk is perceived as a stressful added burden. Other couples say they talk frequently, maybe phoning three or four times from the office, chatting as they organize their day in the morning and again at lunchtime—and then spending time together or with their family in the evening. With some couples, both partners work from home, giving them constant opportunity for interaction.

Through my research, I've seen that the amount of time partners talk—the actual number of minutes or hours—does not always translate into quality of conversation or liveliness of the interchange. Even when couples chat a lot during the day about mundane things—the weekly schedule, what to have for supper, and Suzy's snuffling nose—they are not necessarily discussing anything meaningful to either of them, such as their desires, longings, or dreams. Even everyday things that are important to each of them as individuals, such as a stress at the office, a unique experience, or a simple need for attention, may go unshared when couples have busy schedules and especially if they have young children. It's not possible, or even necessary, to share all your thoughts and feelings or have frequent deep discussions about desires and dreams. However, when couples don't talk often enough about things that are important to them, they lose the special connection that comes from having a thread of communication unique to the two of them.

By implementing Step 2 of this program, you will develop a simple and consistent thread of communication that nurtures your partnership and fosters an environment in which to easily and safely share your everyday experiences, thoughts, and feelings, as well as your passions and dreams.

## How Many Minutes a Day Do You *Really* Talk to Each Other?

Mohammed and Sari are busy professionals with erratic schedules. They have been married for nearly seven years and have an energetic preschool-aged son they take turns caring for with some help from a nanny a few times each week.

When they first approached me to help their troubled relationship, they were frustrated with each other, angry and resentful that their needs were not being met. In their first session, they turned their bodies away from each other, had almost no eye contact, and showed no physical affection. They talked resentfully as though the other person was not even in the room. Sari retreated into silence. Mohammed's talk frequently became heated and verbose. When prompted, they spoke of the early days of their relationship— before having a child and a house in need of remodeling—when they had stimulating conversations about everything from current events to a love of movies and music they shared to career and relationship aspirations. They loved to travel and indulged this passion often. They explored friendships with interesting people who shared their love of art and culture. When I asked them how much time they spent talking each day, they quickly said it was sporadic and depended on their often-conflicting work schedules. When I asked them what they talked about and how these conversations proceeded, they reported that sometimes discussions were "about more superficial things, often smooth, and even had some humor and playfulness," but at other times these discussions "easily deteriorated into disagreement, anger, then silence for hours or days." As a rule, Mohammed and Sari communicated mainly about daily to-do lists and their son.

Mohammed and Sari were cranky and unhappy in this marriage. Like many couples, they had begun to wonder if they had made a mistake in marrying each other. They were in mourning, grieving the loss of their earlier days, with the companionship, rich friendships, and common interests they had obviously shared and thrived on. Their relationship had become a combination Traditional/Roommate Style, and neither was happy with it. They are a prime example of two people who have forgotten they are able to change their situation and feel like victims of their circumstances. They had become devoted parents but had sacrificed their marriage.

Once the initial honeymoon phase has faded and two people have lived together for a few years or once children have come along, a couple spends much less time talking about truly personal and meaningful things. Stresses and demands of daily life become the major focus in many households. Husbands, wives, mothers, fathers, and children come and go with little time to focus on one another. With little opportunity to share more deeply, couples stop getting to know each other. Because we are always growing and changing as individuals, it is easy to drift apart if there is no ongoing thread of communication. This leaves couples more vulnerable to loneliness, depression, anger, and frustration. It also leaves couples seeking attention outside of the relationship.

This is how Sari explained their situation:

> I used to talk and talk and tell him what I wanted and how I was feeling. He'd listen and really showed me he cared. Now he tunes me out. At some point he just seemed to get tired of hearing anything I had to say, and he stopped talking to me about his life. Over the years I've tried every tactic to get him to talk to me—some loving, and some I'm not so proud of. I don't know what happened. I've just given up. I don't have the energy. I don't have much feeling—about anything. I don't know what I want anymore. I don't know how to talk to him. I'm so angry and hurt. I don't know if I even love him. I don't know what I feel.

Many people start to resent and blame their partner rather than identify difficult communication as a problem stemming from lack of steady, meaningful connection. They fail to recognize this as a problem they can solve together. For some men and women, resentment turn into passivity, depression, and withdrawal from their mate; for others, antipathy is expressed through anger, blame, and sometimes disrespectful or abusive language. As you will discover throughout these 10 Steps, while these feelings may be human and normal, they should not be acted on. Instead, you will practice ways of talking to each other from your intention to *partner*, without putting your problems between you. Then you will learn new ways to resolve your problems together.

Mohammed and Sari are an example of how not talking consistently to each other can lead to assumptions and resentments. These resentments are then acted out through increased negative exchanges. When people stop talking and stop having positive interactions (Steps 1 and 2), they end up in a troubled cycle. Using Step 2, talking together regularly and listening carefully to each other, you will avoid these troubles just as Mohammed and Sari learned to do. Like Mohammed and Sari, you both want the same thing—a solid, happy life together.

---

**TIP**: To improve your relationship, agree to develop a thread of consistent and meaningful communication. Begin by scheduling times to talk together regularly and take turns listening to each other about topics that are important to each of you.

---

Talking and listening regularly improves the quality of your interaction. It also gives full attention to the topic that is important to your partner.

In the Big Picture approach, partners are asked to spend twenty to thirty minutes at least every other day, or four times per week, taking turns talking and listening to each other. Each person is allowed roughly half of the time for the partner's undivided attention.

Now, scheduling twenty to thirty minutes every other day to maximize the quality and efficiency of communication might sound clinical. Some feel this conversation would or should happen spontaneously "if he really loved me" or "if she really cared." For other couples, finding the time for a conversation at the end of the day when they are too tired or burned out seems nearly impossible. This resistance is exactly why it's so important to talk together regularly and take turns listening.

When first given this assignment, some couples are so out of practice they don't know what to talk about or how to fill the ten to fifteen minutes allotted to each partner. If this happens to you the first few times, simply share your responses to the exercises at the end of each chapter, and you will have plenty to talk about. If you are having trouble finding time to talk, try creating a schedule like the one that appears on page 49:

## ✚ REHAB TOOLKIT
## Make Time to Talk

Agree to schedule twenty to thirty minutes of conversation, with no interruptions, at least four times each week or every other day. This is a time in which you sit down or take a walk together and talk about something that is important and meaningful to you—not schedules, not the kids, not household errands. Then your partner does the same, talking about something important to him or her while you listen. While you can have some interaction and dialogue, the objective is to actively listen to your partner; to get to know your partner today, in this moment; and to let your partner know more about you by sharing your desires, concerns, goals, and dreams.

Sample week: November 15-22

| Saturday,<br>Nov. 15 | Monday,<br>Nov. 17 | Wednesday,<br>Nov. 19 | Friday,<br>Nov. 21 |
|---|---|---|---|
| a.m. coffee | after kids<br>go to bed | early walk<br>before work | dinner out |
| ✔ | ✔ | ✔ | ✔ |

*Here is a sample check-off system you can create to help you remember to schedule twenty to thirty minutes every other day or four times a week to take turns talking and listening to one another.*

## Talking Creates Dramatic and Ongoing Improvements

Even though couples vary in the amount of time they talk, regular talking and listening nearly always improves the overall quality of the relationship. While Dr. Gottman's research discussed in Chapter 3 shows that a high ratio of positive-to-negative interactions is an essential factor in the longevity of marriages, my observations show that developing a consistent pattern of meaningful communication in any couple is equally important. Both are easy to reintegrate in your relationship; both empower you to quickly nourish your relationship and improve how you feel about yourself and each other.

Couples who . . .

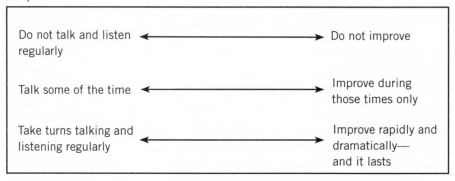

*The above diagram shows how talking and listening can help your relationship.*

So how did implementing this essential step—talking together—affect Mohammed and Sari?

During the first coaching session, we assessed their relationship style, which had deteriorated to Traditional/Roommate. They agreed to stop fighting while they practiced Step 1, increasing the positives between them. They also agreed to begin Step 2 and schedule regular talking and listening time, discussing things that had once been important to them. I told them to do so until they returned for their next session.

Two weeks later, a different couple walked into the room. They were sweet and playful with each other, reporting their progress with a bit of sparkle, humor, eye contact, and touch. Talking had been difficult at first, but they were determined to see if they could learn to partner, and they had been successful in talking at least five of the eight times. At first, they felt shy or unsure of what to say. They decided to share some early childhood memories. Then they talked about what they each loved about their courtship days. Soon Sari was sharing an experience that had made her feel cared about. Mohammed took a risk and talked about how her behavior or tone of voice sometimes really hurt his feelings even though he seldom showed it. They even talked about the dreams of travel and adventure that had been buried.

Mohammed and Sari quickly reported more fun and flow in their lives as they developed a pattern of consistent talking during the next month. They were entertaining friends at a dinner party they created together, planning a bit of travel as a couple for their anniversary, and devoting days to play and family activities with their son. Their heavy work schedules had not changed. As they talked, they began to feel less like Roommates and behave less Traditionally; they began to partner.

During the next few months of coaching, Mohammed and Sari twice experienced what happens when they stop talking regularly and listening to each other. Once the family was sick for two consecutive weeks, and they were lazy about talking meaningfully even though all three were home in bed. They slipped into their more Traditional roles, with Sari waiting on her husband and child even though she was just as ill. Another time, Mohammed brought his unhappiness about work into his marriage, and he stopped talking to Sari about the stress he was feeling at work. They felt like Roommates when this happened. Both times, the old behaviors made them discontented. After the second time this happened, they got it: "We haven't been talking enough!"

Once they fully grasped the "key" they each held to improving their relationship, Mohammed and Sari felt empowered. Together they could easily go from a Traditional/Roommate Style to Big Picture Partnering; they could go from unhappiness to contentment—and even joy—in a matter of minutes, by simply devoting the time to talking meaningfully with each other.

As you continue to table your fights, create more positive feelings, talk together regularly and take turns listening, you and your partner can feel empowered, too.

## Talking Increases Connection

The act of listening to your partner and being listened to validates your existence and the importance of your partnership. It makes you feel "known" and cared about. It is the thread of communication that some call a feeling of connection. Talking sustains and nourishes the opportunity for intimacy in a busy, hectic, and often demanding world. It is nice to truly know your partner deeply, and to have your partner know you.

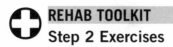

## REHAB TOOLKIT
## Step 2 Exercises

### *Reflections on Your Current Communication*

Reflect for a moment on the amount you and your partner talk to each other each day. How much time is actually focused on the two of you rather than on kids, friends, family, or scheduling the next day's activities? How often do you share something important or take the time to turn off the phone or BlackBerry and really listen to each other, uninterrupted?

How do you feel about your pattern of communication? How has it changed over the years and what do you think has brought about those changes?

Now think for another moment. When would be a good time to spend twenty to thirty minutes alone together? Would it be early or late in the day? Over morning coffee or during an evening walk? After the kids are in bed at night? Will you both be wide awake? Could you possibly do this every other day or four times each week? Do you think it might be difficult to know what to say if you don't talk very much? Might you actually enjoy it?

### *Develop a Thread of Meaningful Communication*

Your joint assignment is to incorporate regular talking and listening into your daily lives. Use the guidelines on the following pages to help you. Some of you may find this very easy; others may find it very challenging. No one is perfect. Some days or weeks will be better than others. What is important is that you start developing a communication pattern with a great deal of consistency.

This week, you can use one regular talking time to share your thoughts about the previous exercise, Reflections on Your Current Communication, and to plan a schedule of regular talking for the rest of the week.

## Regular Talking/Taking Turns Listening

- Schedule twenty to thirty minutes every other day or four times per week as times to talk together.

- Allow no interruptions. Agree not to answer the doorbell or the telephone. Make sure children are either asleep, being cared for by someone else, or if they're older, instructed not to interrupt you.

- If an emergency arises, reschedule your talking time with your partner ASAP.

- If for some reason your partner stands you up, take the time anyway. Use it for reflection, perhaps writing in your notebook about the topic you had chosen to talk about. You can then share the topic with your partner later.

- Each person must talk for ten to fifteen minutes. It is OK to respond a bit or ask questions now and then; however, a guiding principle is to mostly listen to the talking partner.

- Take turns beginning the conversation. When your turn to talk arrives, choose a topic that is important to you. Do not talk about schedules or the kids. If you always talk about work or money, do not talk about these during regular talking time. Challenge yourself to talk about something that is important to you.

- It is not imperative that you agree or disagree. What is essential is to be together, to be willing to share, to open up a little, to be heard, and to do so on a regular basis.

- Try to begin to establish some consistency early on. Don't become discouraged if a few weeks go by before you find your rhythm and establish this regular talking time.

## Chapter 5

# STEP 3:

## Deepen Your Individuality to Strengthen Your Relationship

While you continue to increase the positives between you (Step 1) and integrate regular talking and listening (Step 2), you are about to embark on strengthening and building the "muscles of adulthood."

Everything you know about communicating and caring you learned in childhood. These lessons are a familiar and natural part of your interactions with others, until they are no longer effective and you are forced to learn new ways of communicating and behaving. Becoming aware of these unconscious early patterns is one lesson included in **Big Picture Step 3: Deepen Your Individuality to Strengthen Your Relationship**. The other lesson is to become educated in more effective ways of communicating and interacting with each other. Both lead to more adult interactions and will keep your communication in good shape.

Some of the benefits of communicating and interacting from a solid adult core are

- saying what you mean and meaning what you say;

- having fewer misunderstandings;

- experiencing less defensiveness and fewer fights, less bickering, and fewer flare-ups;

- feeling lighter and having more fun because talking is easier.

Now you may huff and puff and say, "But we *are* adults! We *do* communicate as adults! What can you possibly mean?"

My answer is that you probably do communicate and interact as adults and often very successfully at the office or with your colleagues and friends. On the other hand, you—like many other couples—probably revert to speaking in hurtful ways you are not proud of, or from time to time, you may feel shamed or blamed by your partner. There are unresolved issues you avoid or fight about with no mutual solution. You may have a pattern of squabbling over things that really don't matter, and you can't seem to stop the pattern from happening repeatedly.

The lessons in this chapter will highlight your contribution to this pattern through understanding the parent, child, and adult selves that are unconsciously motivating you. You will reflect on what you need to do to stay in your Adult Self, to strengthen the muscles of your Adult Self, and to take care of your Wounded Child Self that takes over when we are under stress.

I promise that if you both embrace this step of the program, your difficult communications and interactions will quickly change. Differences and disagreements may no longer seem as problematic to talk through. Some previous difficulties may even fall away. You will feel better. You'll have more time and energy to focus on fun and creative pursuits in your life.

## Discovering and Developing Your Adult Self

As you begin this chapter, remember that it requires the participation of two whole, Adult Selves to make a Big Picture Partnership. These whole, healthy Adult Selves bring their entirety to the relationship—wonderfulness and quirks, families and friends, work and hobbies, finances and lifestyle activities, challenges and individuality. Exploring and developing your uniqueness—the characteristics, talents, and values that define who you are as individuals—is the premier task of growing up.

Longitudinal research from a variety of experts has delineated a short list of life activities and attributes that contribute to happy, healthy adulthood. As you strengthen the muscles of your Adult Self, you can balance these characteristics in your life and between the two of you. These attributes include developing

- your self-awareness by spending time in self-reflection;

- a vigorous curiosity about life;

- a balance between your masculine and feminine aspects;

- your ability to empathize with and express compassion for others;

- your enjoyment of close and satisfying relationships;

- a deeper meaning in your life.


By embracing this task of developing and maturing your Adult Self, you become motivated to fully express your uniqueness in the world. This is your creative expression. These are your gifts or talents. This self-expression may be manifest in many ways: how you parent, teach, write, or paint. It may be in the making of wonderful food or how you dress, talk, dance, walk, sing, or play. Think about it: You have the opportunity, and the choice, to express yourself uniquely every moment of every day. It is just like the choice to love. You can hide yourself under a basket, or you can take risks to become just a little more wildly, joyously, fully creative—and thus more fully you.

## How Do You Gain the Characteristics of Happy, Healthy Adults?

A helpful way of teaching couples to distinguish their healthy adult behaviors from unhealthy interactions comes out of Transactional Analysis (TA). TA is a school of psychological thought that developed the idea that within each of us are Parent, Adult, and Child selves. This simple approach to the human personality will

- provide you with an understanding of the responses and reactions that help or hinder your relationships;

- empower you with options to change negative responses to your partner and respond in ways that are appropriate to the situation.


Once you can distinguish your healthy adult behavior from unhealthy conduct, your repertoire of skills, both communicating and interacting, will quickly expand. What made you feel stuck before will change when you have a repertoire of healthy behavioral choices and you learn to speak with clarity. I think of expanding this repertoire of adult behaviors as muscle building;

sometimes we all need a personal trainer to teach us new strategies and keep us on track. Using the Parent/Adult/Child (PAC) model is an integral part of your training, which in turn will help you recognize and change the behavior that hinders your relationship.

In this view of the human personality, we experience one of three basic selves at any one time: the Parent, the Adult, and the Child. The Parent and Child selves each have a positive and an unhealthy, or wounded, aspect that will be further described. Remember, the ultimate goal is to become aware of these selves and to develop a strong Adult Self. When you achieve these goals, you develop emotional flexibility. The more flexible and resilient your personality becomes,

- the more flexible you will be in navigating between these selves;
- the more options you will have in your communications;
- the more you will be able to partner in a healthy way.

## The Parent Self

Carole and Bob, married eleven years, have a natural ability to spread goodwill and warmth to everyone in their lives. Their affection for their rambunctious two-year-old twins, Alec and Tim, is obvious. Everyone would say they are fantastic parents. One parent is always watching over their active boys, gently wiping a runny nose, drying tears, distracting them when they take each other's toys, rocking them when they get sleepy, singing and telling them bedtime stories. Observing Carole and Bob, you'd note they are just as kind to the family pet—a big yellow Lab named Max, who guards over the boys patiently as they crawl all over him—as they are to their children.

Carole and Bob worked hard to develop a strong partnership early in their relationship. When they met, each had prior relationship experiences that made them conscious of wanting to make changes. They knew that if they were to have a long life together they had to talk and make many decisions together. They wanted to be sure their values and priorities were clear and consistent. They would need to not only have fun, but also they would have to resolve differences and go through disappointment and trials just as they would go through wonderful times.

Carole and Bob were aware that being "in love" was wonderful, but it was not enough to make a lasting partnership. They knew that their respective families had both positive and negative role modeling. They wanted to keep the good and learn new ways to interact and communicate, so they would not carry on anything negative. In addition, Carole and Bob also wanted children, so they were highly motivated to become the healthiest, most mature and loving people they could become—for each other and for the children they desired.

You may recognize a similar longing to feel fully mature and effective in your relationship; you may share a desire to model healthy interactions and communications for your children's learning, as well as for your own sense of success. Through the lessons you will learn in this chapter, Bob and Carole mastered Step 4, learning how to distinguish this Adult Self from their Parent and Child selves.

Bob and Carole started their family in their late thirties, so their parents were older, and Carole's needed much attention and physical care. Carole and Bob shared these responsibilities with Carole's three siblings, who commented on how loving Carole and Bob were to Carole's parents. In fact, Bob and Carole were as caring and nurturing toward Carole's parents as they were toward their children, Alec and Tim.

In their roles as caregivers to their children, and now their parents, Bob and Carole acted in their role as positive Parent Selves. The Parent Self has both positive characteristics and negative or unhealthy characteristics. You internalized these characteristics as you observed adult behaviors toward you and around you when you were a child. Early role models may include our parents as well as older siblings, grandparents, aunts, uncles, babysitters, and teachers. As we grow older, the behaviors and attitudes of the parent figures around us are unconsciously internalized, until they seem like "a part of us." They simply feel like your own thoughts, feelings, and behaviors.

If you look at the diagram of the Parent Self, the positive aspects of this state are nurturing and caring, as Bob and Carole were with their parents and kids.

## Some Positive Parent Aspects:

- Nurturing children
- Caring for a sick or elderly people
- Showing affection for animals

These are the way we care for a child, a pet, or very sick or old parents.

In partnering relationships, problems arise when we try to parent our partner. When we do nurture another adult out of the parental state, it typically feels like condescension or being treated like a child. This is different from healthy nurturing or caring for a partner from our Adult Self, which I will describe later in this chapter.

The negative or unhealthy side of the Parent Self is called the Critical Parent. The Critical Parent embodies the characteristics you have internalized that are not only critical, but also shaming, blaming, judging, being self-righteous, or angry. It may be spoken criticism or a silent judgmental vibe. Sometimes giving someone the cold shoulder, showing a look of disgust, rolling the eyes in utter dismay, or even shunning a person for a time demonstrates the Critical Parent. You may recognize this as pointing an angry finger at others or even pointing it at yourself. Carole and Bob's experiences provide an example. In talking about her husband, Carole said,

> *Some Negative or Critical Parent Aspects:*
> - Shaming
> - Blaming
> - Judging
> - Anger
> - Shunning
> - Criticism
> - Self-righteousness

Bob is sometimes his own worst enemy. He's a wonderful man, and he's a perfectionist. I can tell when he's let himself down. He'll become quiet and sullen. Once in a while he'll pick on me or become critical of the twins. It's not usually like him. But it does remind me of how his dad always snaps at his wife—Bob's mom—and talks down to anyone who doesn't follow the old man's rules for how to live life. He sure knows how to make a person feel worthless! I think that's why Bob has become so loving in his own life—not wanting to be like his father in that way. Yet it comes out when he doesn't live up to his own expectations. I'll find out later that he overlooked someone at the office, or that someone he supervises made a mistake and Bob feels he handled it poorly. He can get himself coming and going.

Just like Bob, many people are their own worst Critical Parent—they need no one else to blame them or point a shaming finger at them. They do it to themselves, silently and internally. If you ask Bob how this feels he'd say he feels sullen and self-critical and he goes into shame. He feels like a negative father figure disgusted with himself.

It's best not to spend any time in the Critical Parent state, because it is demeaning, detrimental to self-esteem, and harmful to you and any relationship. Instead, I will show you the benefits and behaviors of developing a strong Adult Self.

✚ **REHAB TOOLKIT**
**Getting to Know My Parent Self**

As you read this section, reflect on your Parent Self and consider, "What behaviors and attitudes did I learn from adults around me as a child, and how do I use them positively (with children, animals, or elderly or sick people in my life) or in negative ways with myself, my partner, and other people around me now?" You may wish to write in your notebook, making two lists that you can expand on in the exercises at the end of this chapter.

## The Child Self

When Bob comes home from work, many evenings he and Carole get down on the living room floor to wrestle and play with their two-year-old boys, who squeal with delight at this physical contact. Carole and Bob delight in the affectionate tussle, laughing and making silly noises right along with their boys. Then they end this little predinner ritual by sprawling out in a circle with each one's head on another one's belly—for belly laughing and giggling until they wind down. Bob said,

> It is such a great way to reconnect and switch gears at the end of a long workday. The boys calm down. My head is no longer at work. Carole and I have touched and hugged, and we've all connected once again. No matter what our days have been like, we are all there together, and it feels great.

The Child Self is frequently referred to as the Inner Child. The positive characteristics of an adult's Inner Child are the playful, joyful, generously loving, sometimes mischievous ways we can be when we feel safe and secure with another person or group of people. Maybe we enter this childlike, innocent, playful state with our children. Sometimes we may get silly or mischievous with our mate or with our friends when we are goofing around. It is wonderful to be playfully childlike when we feel safe and secure with those around us.

The negative experience of the Child Self that we carry inside, even in adulthood, is called the Wounded Child. It is the part of yourself that was hurt by people close to you as a child. It reflects how you responded to being hurt by those you loved. If we investigate the feelings and behaviors of our Wounded Child now as an adult, we find a direct reproduction of what we felt, what we thought, and how we behaved when we were hurt in our childhood. The Wounded Child self does not disappear or go away as you mature. Typically it becomes less pronounced or active as you replace childlike responses with more mature responses. Under stress or in close relationships when your feelings are hurt, the Wounded Child responses often reemerge. Sometimes you may act on them, and other times they may simply be private feelings inside.

## Some Positive Child Aspects:

- Playful
- Joyful
- Mischievous
- Innocent
- Curious
- Generous
- Loving
- Trusting
- Affectionate

Bob talked about how his father's behavior influenced him as a child:

> My dad was a heavy drinker when we were growing up. He was a loving man, but then he could turn on you when he had too much to drink. Because we boys were supposed to be little men, when he yelled at me, I'd try not to show it, but I'd feel like dying on the inside! I never was sure I pleased him, and I always wanted him to be proud of me.

> Now I know I'm hard on myself, and others, sometimes. And when my boss is upset with me or Carole hurts my feelings or doesn't give me enough attention—especially since we've had the twins—once in a while I have to work hard not to shut down and withdraw inside. Neither of them is really like my dad, but I find myself doing the same old behaviors once in a while. I'm working on it.

When we think of the possible responses to being hurt as a child, there is a whole continuum of options. If you have children, observe their behaviors when they are hurt by playmates, siblings, teachers, or even by you as a parent.

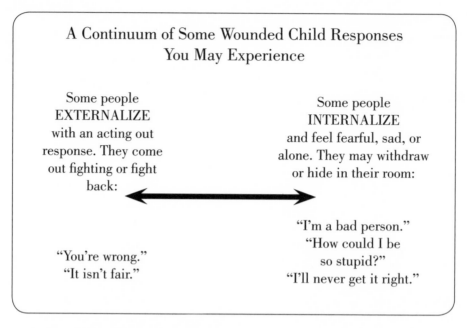

A Continuum of Some Wounded Child Responses
You May Experience

Some people
EXTERNALIZE
with an acting out
response. They come
out fighting or fight
back:

Some people
INTERNALIZE
and feel fearful, sad, or
alone. They may withdraw
or hide in their room:

"I'm a bad person."
"How could I be
so stupid?"
"I'll never get it right."

"You're wrong."
"It isn't fair."

Some children feel very sad or defeated when their feelings get hurt by their parents. They run to their rooms and hide in the closet, or may pull the covers over their heads. They may cry. They may have thoughts about how bad they are, how alone they feel. Some children whose feelings are hurt may come out kicking, screaming, and hollering. To be hurt makes them mad, and they want to lash out. They may think the other person is "unfair" or wrong or bad. Sometimes people describe responding with sadness as a young child, then lashing out angrily as they entered adolescence. Still other children simply don't move when their feelings are hurt. They shut down and "go away" inside while their body stays "present." They may be feeling sadness or defeat—or anger and resentment.

Bob's shutdown and self-critical hurt Child Self may appear similar to the sullenness Carole observes when he internalizes his father's Parent Self, judging and blaming himself. To the outside observer the Critical Parent and Wounded Child selves may be indistinguishable. For example, tough words can be your Critical Parent or your hurt, angry child speaking.

The way you will know is by going inside and assessing whether you feel sad, angry, hurt, or vulnerable. On the other hand, you may feel judgmental and critical like a self-righteous, angry, and blaming parent. When Bob is in his Wounded Child self, he experiences feeling small, feeling little. He does not experience feeling critical or tough like his dad. It is your inner state, your inner experience that gives you the clue to which self is operating. As you complete the following exercise, make note of how you distinguish your Critical Parent Self from your hurting Child Self.

✚ **REHAB TOOLKIT**
## Getting to Know My Child Self

Reflect on your Child Self as you continue to read and write in your notebook. Answer these questions: "What did I do when I was hurt as a young child?" (Examples of behaviors may be standing still but withdrawing inside, running and hiding, kicking and hollering, or some variation.) "What did I feel when I was hurt as a child?" (Examples may include feeling angry, full of rage, sad, confused, devastated, shamed, withdrawn, shutdown, and so on.) Also ask yourself: "What was I thinking when I was hurt as a child?" (Thoughts might be, "I feel so bad, or stupid. I should have known better, how dumb. It's not fair. They are not fair. They are wrong. If only they knew the truth about me. I'm a good person. They think I'm bad and I'm not. They are bad, or wrong, or mean, or to blame.")

Be sure to answer all three questions about your behaviors, your feelings, and your thoughts, especially when you were less than eight years old. If you do not have specific memories, recall a sense of what happened, a pattern of your responses. Then ask yourself, "How do I react similarly in my behaviors, feelings, and thoughts when my partner (or anyone else) hurts my feelings now? How are my behaviors, feelings, and thoughts similar?" You might even reflect on how old you feel inside. This is often a first clue to whether you are in your Child Self; you will feel very young and possibly vulnerable and sad or frustrated and mad.

## The Adult Self

Your Adult Self is the expansive, healthy space or state in which you, as an adult, interact. The Adult Self is spacious and becomes increasingly flexible as you develop your muscles and repertoire of behaviors and communications. The Adult Self has a breadth of thoughts, feelings, actions, and communication. Within the spaciousness, flexibility, and self-acceptance of adulthood, you know and accept your strengths and weaknesses, you discriminate between what you like and don't like. As a healthy adult, you know what you know, what you don't know, and where and when to look for information, help, or advice. As a healthy adult, you are not too humble and you are not too arrogant. You are not too lethargic, neither are you too manic. You have a range of feelings—from love to dislike, anger to acceptance, sorrow to joy, and so on—but you do not let your emotions run your life. They are part of your everyday experience, but they are not to be thrown around or indulged in at anyone else's expense. There is a limit beyond which thoughts, actions, words, and experiences become too extreme or are out of the adult bounds. When they are out of the adult bounds we have tipped into the Critical Parent or Wounded Child self.

Some people react negatively when they think of becoming "adult" or "mature." They want to cling to the vestiges of childhood and maybe even childish behaviors. They misunderstand true adulthood, which is not limiting or stifling. In fact, it is freeing because it encompasses so much of one's life experiences and learning. Most mature adults are far less self-conscious, self-doubting, or concerned with petty things than they were while growing up or in their early adult years. Maturity can bring a lightness of heart and the beginnings of wisdom, so imagine that the Adult Self is spacious! There is room for a great breadth of feelings and behaviors. The edges of your Adult Self help you determine what is healthy or unhealthy. Going beyond these edges lets you know you are too manic or too "in the pits" with depression. As a healthy adult, you know when you are too full of anger and rage or too silent and withdrawn. Caring and loving from your Adult Self is naturally generous and openhearted without any game playing or manipulation or need for payback. You can even be playful and light-hearted as an adult. Most people who cling to childish ways or who refuse to mature do so at the expense of others. They "act out" their emotions when they want to, never taking others into account. Healthy, mature adults know when to work and when to play. They know when to care for others and when to rest and care for themselves.

---

**TIP:** When two strong, resilient Adult Selves connect and communicate, their creativity, intimacy, and satisfaction are enhanced. As we mature, this healthy Adult Self is the state we should strive to be in most of the time when we interact with other adults—especially with our partner. The only exceptions are when both adults are feeling playful, young, and safe with each other, or when one is in a nurturing Parent Self and interacting with a child, elderly person, someone who is ill, or a pet.

---

In learning to think, feel, and behave as your Adult Self, there are two strategies to become aware of:

- Avoid bouncing back and forth between your Child Self and Parent Self, so you don't bypass your Adult Self.

- Allow your Adult Self to care for your Child Self, so that you don't look to your partner (and others) to do so.

## ✚ REHAB TOOLKIT
## Getting to Know My Adult Self

Reflect on your Adult Self. When are you most in your Adult Self? The readings in this chapter should help you distinguish your Adult inner state from your Parent and Child Selves. Notice each of your selves throughout the coming days and weeks and ask yourself, "How easy or difficult is it to get back to my Adult Self when I am feeling like a Critical Parent or Wounded Child?" When you can smoothly and easily get back to your Adult Self, you will be consciously in charge of yourself, rather than your Wounded Child or Critical Parent being in charge of you!

## How to Avoid Bypassing Your Adult Self

Once we become aware of the three selves within us, we feel best when we're being our Adult Self. We realize that we've overcome the hurtful parts of childhood, so why continue to revisit them by choice? Besides, the Critical Parent Self just isn't very nice to be around.

As you complete the exercises at the end of this chapter and become more aware of your internal selves, you may notice just how much time you actually spend being the Critical Parent or the Wounded Child. When I ask couples to nonjudgmentally observe their parent/adult/child selves for a week or two, many of them are astounded to discover how much time they spend as the Wounded Child and how often they bounce back and forth between the Wounded Child and the Critical Parent, feeling hurt and sad in the Wounded Child Self, then beating themselves up from the Critical Parent Self, and then feeling bad once again as a Wounded Child. They discover that they don't even require an outside person to be hurtful and critical; their own Critical Parent Self can induce the Wounded Child state—all within themselves!

You may find you have this pattern of bypassing your Adult Self at times and reverting to your Critical Parent or Wounded Child. Alternatively, you may find that when you do become your Adult Self, your repertoire of behaviors and verbal responses is small and not very strong—like muscles that are seldom used. Big Picture Partnering and conversations with your partner will enable you to exercise your "muscles" as you develop your Adult Self. In addition, practicing all 10 Steps in this book will give your Adult Self a larger, more flexible set of tools, skills, behaviors, and responses you can use for a lifetime.

Every adult I have worked with has at least a small Adult Self repertoire. You may easily slip into your repertoire around colleagues, coworkers, friends, or new acquaintances. We all use our best adult behavior in public; it is in our private, most personal relationships—with romantic partners and family—that all of our Wounded Child and Critical Parent buttons are pushed and we forget to stay adult.

It is the task of maturing to grow your Adult Self and to spend almost all of your time interacting from within it. If you discover you have weak adult "muscles," start by identifying the muscles that you do have. Then look around for positive adult role modeling. How do other adults behave, interact, and communicate when they are at their best? A key phrase I like to offer people is to always behave with "grace and dignity." Everyone immediately understands grace, dignity, and respect. These concepts summarize and encompass the essence of the Adult Self.

## ✚ REHAB TOOLKIT
## One Way to Build the Muscles of Adulthood

When you find yourself in your Wounded Child or Critical Parent self and you are unsure of what an Adult Self might do in that situation, one clue is to go inside and ask yourself the following important question: How would a normal, healthy adult, behaving with grace and dignity, act in this situation?

In addition, I recommend reading about healthy adult development. Talk to friends. Find a mentor or coach. Observe and interact with other people you admire. Read biographies and autobiographies of people you admire for their grace, their dignity, and the respect they inspire. Participate in your church or community. Give to others who are less fortunate. Gravitate to people and activities that challenge your thinking and your emotional and spiritual growth. All of these exercise the muscles of healthy adulthood.

## ✚ REHAB TOOLKIT
## Developing Your Adult Self

Reflect on what you are doing to grow, learn, and develop your Adult Self. Make a list of books you are reading, people you turn to, and activities you participate in that stretch and strengthen your adult muscles. Turn to page 56 at the beginning of this chapter, and review the list of life attributes that make people healthy and happy in their lives. What are you doing to achieve each characteristic on your list? What would you like to improve or work on in the coming year or two, as you become a strong adult and a solid Big Picture Partner? Remember, as you strengthen your Adult Self,

- the more flexible you will be in navigating between your selves;

- the more options you will have in your communications;

- the more you will be able to partner in a healthy way.

---

If you have not yet learned enough adult behaviors and responses, it is not too late, regardless of your age. If both you and your partner work to strengthen your Adult Selves, you will have the inner strength—the adult "muscles"—to tackle the Big Picture adventure as you continue to build your rock-solid partnership.

## Handling Emotions as an Adult

Sometimes your Adult Self may need something as simple as a refresher in table manners or social graces to feel competent in the larger world. Sometimes your Adult Self may need something more complex such as new ways to communicate with your boss or a coworker. Sometimes we need to know the boundaries of sexuality or how to stay adult in heated discussions or arguments. Trying to resolve stressful grown-up matters—your partner's insensitive behavior or your hurt feelings when your partner seems unaware of your needs—is futile when one or both of you become childish or critical.

According to TA, our Parent, Adult, and Child selves always exist. We carry each within us forever. They do not grow up or go away. Even if you successfully strengthen your adult muscles, in stressful or trigger situations you may still revert to the behaviors of a Wounded Child or the Critical Parent. The adult emotions are appropriate and effective. The Wounded Child emotions are valid as well; they are just not very effective in getting what you want and need in your adult life. The Critical Parent should be avoided altogether.

In couple relationships, if one or both individuals try to have their needs met when in a Wounded Child state, the result can be damaging and frustrating.

Ivan, married four years to Marlene, talked about how the Child and Parent selves play out in their relationship at times:

> When I'm feeling vulnerable, I sure can't show it around Marlene. She expects me always to be strong and lectures me about all the ways I could improve my situation. I end up feeling like she's trying to be my mother. I know she doesn't want this either, but it leaves me feeling unmanly, and extremely angry with her in the long run. She says she feels trapped by my behavior when I'm needy like that and doesn't know how to respond in a positive way. She tries, but we both lose out.

Learning to stay in their Adult Selves has improved Ivan and Marlene's situation immensely.

Penny, who has been living with Mike for nine months, said the two of them are also grappling with the parent/child predicament:

> I feel so out of sorts these days and I don't think Mike knows what to do, so he just goes silent on me. I cry and make a scene when he's not home on time, and I miss him or am worried about him. I feel so immature, yet I can't keep myself from acting this way. I know everything is OK between us, but moving in together is more stressful than I could have imagined.

Jerome and Julia have come up with their own strategies for staying adult. Said Julia,

> It's taken a few years, but now when one of us is feeling down, or hurt, or little, the other one tries to stay adult and just listens until the feelings subside.

Jerome added,

> I think we are also both better at nurturing our own wounds, talking to our friends, or going for a walk or run when we are initially hurt. Then we come

back and talk later when we feel able to talk more calmly. Sometimes, by then, the feelings have gone away. If not, we quickly clear the air.

According to TA, we need to become our own best caregivers. You are the adult who now needs to nurture your own inner child. Looking to your partner for "parenting" will lead to inequality and imbalance in your relationship.

Your Adult Self needs to take responsibility for your Child Self. You need to let the adult part listen to this child or take yourself "out to play" and give yourself attention when your feelings have been wounded and the hurt is not resolved. If your Adult Self does not protect and care for the child inside you, it is like having a three-year-old in your care and walking away when the child is hurting. If you let your Critical Parent take over, it's like punishing a small child with shame or blame. It is important that you learn to care for your inner child from a loving adult place so you don't inappropriately lay this burden on your mate. Examples:

- Your healthy Adult Self knows the old habits you may fall into when you visit your family. The Adult Self can visit your extended family and leave your Child Self at home—safe and protected.

- Your healthy Adult Self knows how to get through a difficult or heated discussion when your Child Self feels afraid or acquiesces out of fear or uncertainty.

- Your healthy Adult Self knows how to stand up for yourself in an assertive way when someone is bullying you.

- While your Child Self may not know how to say no, your healthy Adult Self can do so when appropriate.

- Your healthy Adult Self can take your Child Self out for ice cream or comfort you when you need a good cry.

- Your healthy Adult Self knows how to have good, intimate sex. The Adult Self also knows not to engage in sex if you are feeling little, hurt, or needy.

- Your healthy Adult Self can remind your Child Self that making mistakes is part of learning, that there's nothing to be ashamed of, and that you'll be able to do better next time.

Such tasks are much too big for a three- or four-year-old. They are not too big for an adult.

In the following exercises, you will continue to identify your Parent, Child, and Adult selves. Incorporate your individual reflections from earlier exercises throughout the chapter. Becoming acquainted with your responses will help you to stay positive with your partner and strengthen the adult/adult interactions between you.

Take your time and complete these exercises thoroughly on your own. Later you will come together to share your discoveries.

Once you become fully aware of your three selves, change will come more easily. The main task is to ask yourself is, "Am I using these selves wisely? How do I revert to the Critical Parent or the Wounded Child when I am under stress? How does reverting affect my interactions with people and especially my partnership? Does my Adult Self need some muscle building? Which characteristics of my Adult Self do I need to work on?"

As you will be identifying both positive and negative characteristics in yourself and your partner, try to remain nonjudgmental, yet truthful.

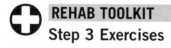

## REHAB TOOLKIT
## Step 3 Exercises

### Positive and Negative Parent Selves

These exercises will help you identify the times in your life when you think or behave as the positive or negative parent—or when you feel your partner, or others, are behaving in this way. Refer back to the lists of positive and negative parent aspects on pages 58 and 59 to help you.

First make a list of the times when you find yourself being the positive, or nurturing, Parent Self. Identify times you experience being a Parent Self with your partner. Ask yourself if you are expressing the positive Parent Self appropriately. When might it be inappropriate to express this self with your partner—and how does being a positive Parent Self have an impact on your relationship?

Identify what you say and do when you are your negative Parent Self. When do you revert to the negative Parent Self, and how does this affect your relationship? How does your partner respond when you are being a Critical Parent? Ask yourself, "When I've used Critical Parent words and actions with my partner, what dynamic does it produce? Is this the result I want?"

Now look at times when your partner has pointed a Critical Parent finger at you, verbally or nonverbally. When does this typically happen in your relationship? How does receiving the Critical Parent treatment make you feel? How do you respond? Do you remain calm? Do you feel little and sad? Do you become angry and rebellious? What impact does giving or receiving Critical Parent treatment have on your relationship?

Sometimes we are our own worst Critical Parent. Explore when you are critical of or shaming, blaming, angry, or judging yourself. Ask yourself, "How do I feel when I am being the Critical Parent and pointing a finger at myself?"

Take some time to identify all the triggers or stressors that seemingly cause you to revert to any of the negative or Critical Parent behaviors, such as speaking angrily, shaming yourself or shaming your partner, or blaming or criticizing yourself or your partner. Again, ask yourself, "Is this the result I want?"

## Joyful and Wounded Child Selves

These exercises will help you identify the times in your life when you think or act like the joyful or Wounded Child—or when you feel your partner, or others, are acting this way.

Focus first on your joyful child experience. Ask yourself, "How does my joyful Child Self act when I feel safe? How do I play and express humor, laughter, mischievousness, and joy? How often do my partner and I interact and play as Child Selves? Is this often enough?"

Now, focusing on the Wounded Child, ask yourself, "How did I react when I was hurt as a child (before the age of eight or nine years)?" Think about your initial response. You may have had a secondary response within minutes, but it is the first response that is most important. Explore what you did "on the outside." Did you kick, scream, cry, look blank or impassive, run to your room, or hide?

Next, consider what you were thinking and feeling "on the inside." You may have felt sad, hurt and confused, angry, or even enraged. In either case, what were you telling yourself? Was it "I'm such an awful, stupid person!" or "It's so unfair. They are wrong or stupid to treat me this way!"?

As you contemplate your childhood responses, think about whether or how you might subtly replicate them today when you feel hurt, shamed, blamed, or punished or when someone is angry or misunderstanding you. You'll probably discover your Wounded Child responses hiding in adult clothing. Write about how these responses affect your relationship. When you act from your Wounded Child Self, do you get the results you want with your partner?

## Your Adult Self

These exercises are meant to help you identify your current adult strengths and to explore ways to expand on them, so you and your partner interact from your Adult Selves most of the time.

First, using your notebook, write these words at the top of a blank page: *What I notice about my Adult Self*. Then slowly think over all of your relationships. Think about how you behave with your coworkers, friends, parents, siblings, and partner. Make a list of six of these people, including your partner and at least one parent (living or deceased). Under each person's name, identify the adult qualities you show around this person. (For example, your partnership may challenge you to be your all-around best. In your position at work, you may be calmly in charge and coach those you manage with warmth and wisdom. Around your parents, you may show compassion and caring as they age. A good friend may bring out your playfulness while a sibling who looks up to you may draw on your mentoring abilities.)

Then stop and reflect on these six lists. When is it most difficult to stay adult around each of these people? Make another list of an additional three adult characteristics or qualities (greater patience, more compassion, a willingness to talk through conflicts, less defensiveness, more tolerance, etc.) that you would like to increase in each of these relationships. Notice if the list for your partner is similar or different from those for the other people in your life. Ask yourself, "Am I bringing my Adult Self equally to all of my relationships, or is it more challenging to do this with my partner?"

Also ask yourself how you respond in any of these relationships: "Do I bypass my Adult Self and instead become the Critical Parent? Do I then beat myself up, become the Wounded Child, feel hurt or angry, and then beat myself up again? When do I do this? Under what circumstances do I bypass my Adult Self?" The pattern might seem a little like a boomerang from Critical Parent to Wounded Child.

As a way of expanding your adult behavioral repertoire, think about the people around you. Who consistently acts in ways you admire and want to emulate? Look for a variety of people at work, among your friends, your neighborhood or faith community, and among celebrities. You may even think back to positive role models you had as a youngster, in high school, or in college.

In addition, you may list all the current professionals—advisors, coaches, teachers, and mentors—who could help you develop adult "muscles."

Again, taking a blank page in your notebook and contemplating everything you have learned about your Parent, Child, and Adult selves, answer the following question: "What do I need to do to strengthen my Adult Self?"

Then highlight four or five things you can do to help yourself to stay adult or expand your adult repertoire. Make specific notes and agreements with yourself about what you intend to do to strengthen your Adult Self in the coming days, weeks, and months. (You might start with your partner and work on listening without judgment when he or she talks to you. At work, you might decide to become more of a leader and offer to teach someone a skill that you know. If you wait for others to phone you, you might decide to call one or two acquaintances or friends and go out for coffee to practice reaching out.)

### Letting Your Adult Self Care for Your Joyful and Wounded Child

As your Adult Self becomes strong and confident, it will become easier to care for the Wounded Child inside, so the child feels nurtured and does not sabotage your relationship. You should become aware of how you behave when you are feeling joyful or hurt, and then nurture yourself appropriately. Most of our Child Self's needs are small and manageable—to be loved, acknowledged, and given attention. Ask yourself the following question: "How do I nurture myself?"

Now write five or six ways you can nurture yourself when you feel a little down. Forms of nurturing might include a long, hot, relaxing bath, a well-prepared and delicious meal, listening to music, or a conversation with a close friend.

Now ask yourself, "How do I fulfill my Child Self's need to play?" This could be a romp in the yard with your dog, a jog around the lake, a pillow fight with your older sister, a trip to the movies, or creating a piece of art. Some people enjoy making ice cream or playing golf. What would satisfy your Child Self's needs?

As part of your self-care while you practice this step, identify what your inner child might like to do for fun or relaxation. Then, provided it is not harmful or prohibitively expensive, do it. Care for this part of yourself by giving yourself enough time for play, rest, or creative pursuits.

Make a list of all the things you can do to care for your inner child when your feelings are hurt. What do you most need and want when you are feeling bad? How can you give yourself special care when your feelings are wounded? Taking care of yourself in this way is very important, because if you don't, you will expect your partner to take care of your Wounded Child.

See if your inner child and your Adult Self can create a strong relationship. You will feel more cared for and nurtured because you are directly in control of providing this Adult care of your Wounded Child feelings and can do so at any time. In addition, your Adult Self will be available to relate to your partner more often, without the hurt feelings of the Wounded Child interfering.

### Talking with Your Partner about Your Parent, Child, and Adult Selves

Once the two of you have done this private reflecting and have thought of ways to strengthen your Adult Selves, come together as partners. Take turns talking and listening to each other as you describe what you are learning about your own ability to stay adult and about what stressors trigger you to revert to the Critical Parent and/or Wounded Child.

Share what you have discovered about your childhood responses to being hurt. Talk about how you see yourself reverting to these patterns in your relationship. Describe one or two things you plan to do to stay adult with each other.

Your task as partners in this exercise is mainly to listen nonjudgmentally. One way to do this is to notice anytime you catch yourself acting from a Critical Parent or Wounded Child place. You quickly say, "Oops, there I go again. Let me stop and start over." As the partner, you'd speedily agree and move on.

## Chapter 6

# STEP 4:

## Discover the Depth of Your Commitment

When a partnership is thriving, commitment comes easily. During stressful times, being fully and consistently dedicated may feel more challenging. Commitment may come easily for you. However, for some of you, practicing the initial steps of this program may have been challenging because your commitment was fraught with hurt, anger, confusion, or disappointment when you picked up this book. Continuing to put your fights aside and increase the positive (Step 1), developing a regular thread of communication (Step 2), and communicating from your Adult Self (Step 3) will change how you feel about yourself and eventually, about each other. **Big Picture Step 4: Discover the Depth of Your Commitment** will teach you why it is important to be fully committed to yourself, each other, and your relationship at all times, and it will teach you the importance of protecting the relationship you value—even when you go through tough times.

When a couple is fully committed to each other and their relationship, the commitment creates safety. Commitment allows you both to trust that your partner will not leave or abandon you when times are tough. It allows you to trust that your partner is pledging 100 percent. Conscious commitment that is also stated aloud—especially during tough or stressful times—reaffirms your devotion and reassures your partner that you are making the necessary changes together.

As you learn Step 4, you will

- read stories about couples navigating change through many phases of their relationships and learn what threatened to tear them apart and what brought them closer together;

- reflect upon formal commitment and daily commitment;

- investigate ways you may undermine commitment from within your relationship;

- learn about ways to protect your relationship from outside pressures.

## What Do We Mean by *Commitment*?

A commitment is a pledge, promise, oath, vow, or agreement given in trust. In a relationship, it is typically a promise of loyalty, fidelity, faithfulness, compassion, and companionship. Commitment to a relationship before marriage or without a ceremony is a private affirmation of the love, harmony, bond, understanding, and desire two people have to build a relationship together. When two people marry, the commitment becomes a public vow, a promise made in the presence of family and friends, sanctioned by God or the state, to create a life together "till death do us part."

### Formal Commitment

There are times to make a formal commitment—or recommitment—to each other, to your relationship, and to the Big Picture future you are building. In this chapter's exercises, you will both have an opportunity to reflect on and make a conscious statement or reaffirmation of your commitment. You may have already done this through an engagement, a marriage, a commitment ceremony, or a renewal of your vows. Even so, take the opportunity this week to make or reinforce that vow. It is a promise to you and to each other.

### Daily Commitment

Another way of showing your commitment is through your daily interactions. Commitment is implied in every action, agreement, and communication as you build your Big Picture Partnering universe, where two whole individuals work to satisfy both individual and mutual needs, desires, and goals. You will become aware of how ongoing dedication is integral to everything you do.

As you develop a strong consciousness of this step of the program, you will notice that your steadfastness is naturally reaffirmed through your everyday interactions and behaviors.

## Challenges to Our Commitments

Some years ago, National Public Television aired a series of interviews with couples that had been together for forty, fifty, or sixty years. In this documentary, each couple related the trials and delights of their long marriage. They talked about their various stages, events, and memories. Some were humorous and playful as they spoke. Others poignantly revealed touches of old pain. One couple almost grudgingly talked of staying together out of convenience and necessity. Others revealed a rich companionship, friendship, and appreciation—a deep and enduring love—that had grown out of the life they had created together.

In this documentary, all of the couples had married and committed at a time when commitment was a strong societal value and expectation. Most of them did not question their vows, and if they did, it was not until they were much older and divorce was more prevalent. When these couples were young, most people expected to marry and raise children. Couples came together not only for love, but also for survival and security; for them, economic stability and raising good, healthy children were very important. They wanted happiness, but they did not always expect it as the primary value or priority. Those married prior to the 1960s generally had a long-term vision of being together and did not consider divorce if they struggled for a time.

If we look at the divorce rate as well as the number of cohabitants who break up today, it is apparent that neither a personal nor a public declaration of commitment is enough to hold many relationships together. Almost 50 percent of marriages end in divorce, and 56 percent of cohabitants eventually separate. Today the motivations for marriage, or for any romantic commitment, are much more varied. Happiness, compatibility, and fulfillment of mutual wants and desires are high on the list of expectations. So when these factors are unfulfilled due to challenges of long-term relating and everyday life, commitment to the relationship is often challenged as well. If people aren't happy for a time—for any reason, large or small—they often question the entire relationship.

Long-term relationships require steady nurturance, continuous affirmation, and commitment. It is joyful to be committed during the honeymoon and the smooth periods of a relationship. However, in any long-term relationship our devotion is challenged at various times. It may be challenged by an event as

77

disruptive and painful as an affair, by the pressures of children or two careers, or even by boredom. Factors such as financial stress, moving, poor health, demanding schedules, or in-laws and extended family may also challenge your commitment.

One couple I've worked with on and off since they were dating has had a relationship filled with many joys and just as many stresses. Together for almost nine years and married for six years, Donna and David experienced the joys of falling passionately in love and sharing a strong sense of life purpose that included being together and creating a thriving relationship and family. Together they had also built a successful business that allowed Donna time with her young sons and David the excitement of training leaders throughout the world. Donna and their two beautiful preschool-aged sons often travel with David to foreign countries where they meet interesting people. In their early forties, both Donna and David share conscious aspirations to do good work and impact the world with their inspiring message, as well as through philanthropy and volunteering, as they grow older.

On the other hand, Donna and David have also navigated the murky waters of premarital infidelity and alcohol addiction. In the early stages of building their business, they suffered bankruptcy, the consequences of which they still feel in minor ways. During this same time, Donna suffered the illness and subsequent death of her sister from cancer. She also experienced post-partum depression following each of her son's births. David is high energy and demanding. He gets angry when Donna is not "at the top of her game" along with him. David's work is exciting, but it takes him away from home nearly half of each month. At times, Donna must pack up the family to accompany him on the business trips while their sons are still young and not in school.

Donna and David have been consciously committed to partnering since their dating years. Neither of them would rate their relationship as Traditional, Merged, or Roommate, except when they go through a transition—such as bankruptcy or having children or any of the other times described. With every challenge, however, this couple has sought to renew and revitalize their Big Picture Partnership. They would be the first to admit they are not perfect, but they want to get better. They also renew their commitment to each other and to their marriage on a daily basis. As Donna explained,

> Whether we are together or apart, no matter where we are in the world on any given night, we always say we are committed to our marriage out loud to each other: "I choose to be married to you today." Sometimes this isn't easy

because one or the other of us may feel angry or depressed, making one of us ambivalent. But we reaffirm our desire to make this relationship work in spite of how difficult it is that day.

David added,

Even when I am mad at her, I love Donna more than anything. I have this vision of how good it is sometimes and how good we can make it if we are both doing the work. We have an incredible life. We have so many blessings not shared by many others on the planet. Saying, "I want to be married to you today. I choose to be married to you today," keeps me in the moment and working through the tough stuff, and it makes the good stuff even more fantastic.

---

**TIP:** A commitment is an agreement that we fully embrace, embody, and act on at all times. During stressful times, commitment may feel difficult or challenging to you. During these times, ask yourself each morning, "Am I WILLING to be here today? Am I willing to do my part fully and generously even though I may not 'feel' like it?" Your WILL—like will power, willingness, conviction, yearning, wish—will allow you to act on your heart's desire, even when you may not "feel like it" or want to.

---

To build a rock-solid and satisfying Big Picture Partnership means that you must commit—and sometimes recommit—not only to each other and to your relationship, but also to the Big Picture: an evolving long-term relationship that the two of you create over the years.

## Commitment Through the Many Phases of Relating

One of the delights of life is that people change. They grow and naturally evolve through the appropriate developmental stages of their teens, twenties, thirties, forties, and for some, all the way through their nineties. Any enduring, intimate relationship needs to evolve over time to keep it vital and fresh. For all couples, each new phase can be like a new "relationship within a relationship," from the honeymoon to the empty nest and the creativity of later life. Each developmental phase poses a challenge to your commitment to each other and to your relationship.

The following sampling of couples across the lifespan represent changes you may experience as you move through many life stages together. Such transitions may be desired and exciting, but they are stressful nonetheless. Their commitment to each other and their relationship became an anchor for each of these couples during times of transition and change. It can become an anchor for you.

Jorge, twenty-three and married six months to Martina, is headed into law school this fall. As Jorge has taken on the commitments of marriage, partnering, and law school, he's not as happy-go-lucky as he was during their courtship. Martina, his twenty-two-year-old bride, noted how much he was changing, almost overnight:

> He's given up going out and drinking with the boys on weekends. He's much more concerned about getting our new house and finances in order so he can study this fall. He's even treating me differently—mainly for the better. I like the changes, but my head is spinning. He's not the light-hearted guy I met two years ago. He's talking to me like a real adult all of a sudden—sharing his plans and dreams about school and his future. He keeps asking me how I feel about everything, and what I need while he's studying so hard. I guess I'd better start figuring this out so we can work together on it, instead of just feeling nervous, or left out.

Retirement is another big change. Beth was concerned about her fifty-nine-year-old husband, Marvin, to whom she's been married for nearly thirty years:

> Marvin's getting near retirement, and his company may even offer him early severance just to ease their workforce. I think he's afraid and doesn't know what he's going to do. He's become quiet and withdrawn these last six months. We try to talk about it, but it's difficult. One hopeful thing—he said he was thinking of taking some carpentry classes at the vocational school nearby starting in a month. He's always been a great carpenter, and we both know plenty of people who need handyman services. He deserves to slow down and do something he'd really enjoy. And, I'd love for us to get an RV to go on road trips around the country!

Liz and Herbert represent another life stage. Liz, widowed for twelve years, is a sparkly seventy-nine-year-old with lovely white hair. She loves to ballroom dance and has become deeply involved with Herbert, eight years her junior and also widowed. Right now they have no issues, no history or baggage. They play and learned about partnering to keep it that way. They talked about marriage, and Liz was considering the changes she'll be facing if she accepts:

> You know, when I was younger I would have been much more cautious. But one never knows how much time they've got left. My attraction to Herbert is very different than with my husband. But then, we raised a family, grew a business, and made a full life, until Sam died of a heart attack at sixty-eight—so young. It took me almost five years to get my life reoriented, and now I have. Dancing has been great exercise, a social outlet, and then there is Herbert! So many men my age are "old," and I'm not! He's able to keep up with me. I think he's a keeper!

Liz and Herbert looked at each other fondly—then Herbert spoke up:

> I think she's a keeper, too. We have such a good time together. We could just both go on living alone and doing our separate lives, but we think it might be more fun to do the next phase together! I think her kids and mine are having an eye-opening experience as they see us so happy, but they are becoming quite supportive.

Like people, relationships need to change. Both internal factors and external circumstances cause changes in an individual or relationship. Often relationships change because of things a couple is trying to accomplish during a particular stage of life. Ellen, thirty-four, is less concerned about her deeply engaging career these days. She and Mike, married five years, are trying to get pregnant. They'd like to have two children before she turns forty. Here's what Mike was thinking about:

> Now that my career is finally stabilized and I'm making a good income, we figure we'd better get going on the baby thing or it may be too late. I had a hard time thinking about it until I landed this good job and finally felt successful—like all men are supposed to feel. I know it's kind of stupid in this liberal day and age, but feeling successful as a man is still important. We both enjoy our careers, but Ellen feels she can always reenter the work force full-time later on. Women in their forties and fifties—and even sixties—are having blossoming careers in this day and age! Especially now that everyone is living so long.

Ellen added,

And men are more likely to want to work in the garden or play with the grandchildren when they get older. I'm actually looking forward to that time. But first, I guess we have to have the babies!

Some change is thrust upon us. Peg and Jim, married fourteen years, in their early- to mid-forties with two preadolescent, sports-minded sons, were suddenly taking care of two generations: their children and Peg's parents, who were in their eighties and struggling:

Dad's Alzheimer's has become so much worse that Mom can't care for him anymore. She's getting tired, so we have recently found a home that will accommodate both their needs—Dad's in an apartment with twenty-four-hour care, and Mom's in her own apartment nearby. We are trying to take turns visiting at least three to four times a week. It's a handful with the boys' baseball, hockey, and other activities.

Expressing the Big Picture Partnering they value, Jim added,

Yeah, sometimes we feel a bit squeezed in the middle, but I don't think we'd choose to do it any other way. We just have to make sure we have time for each other, or our relationship will suffer.

Sometimes change is exciting, and sometimes it is scary because of the unknown. Either way, without change, we grow bored. A strong commitment to each other and to your relationship—and a conscious recommitment whenever you are going through a major change—will help the two of you trust each other and the rock-solid stability of your partnering. Commitment prepares and equips you for the dreams and fun things you can create as well as for the challenges that life is sure to bring.

---

**TIP:** Ongoing and conscious commitment prepares you for action and invests your relationship with power and strength—because you are facing the change together. You can count on each other and your partnering no matter what happens.

---

## Love Is a Work in Progress

In the classic book, *The Road Less Traveled*, M. Scott Peck writes about enduring love. Peck speaks of the mature discipline and quiet care required to make a long-term commitment thrive. In this view, love becomes an action verb. Active loving can involve the simplest of things—I'll-make-your-bed-for-you, let-me-give-you-a-hug-when-you-are-down, and let's-make-love-even-with-our-wrinkles moments. Long-term love is an action—not just a physical chemistry or a short-term feeling of falling. It can be romantic and passionate, but it is so much more than that. It is a work in progress, much like a beautiful work of art that takes months or even years to create. When a painter is laying colors on the canvas day after day, mixing paints on a palette, scratching and rubbing the surface, and adding more layers, sometimes the canvas looks downright awful—maybe even like a mistake. Nevertheless, after perseverance, the hidden tones start to shine through, the richness and depth affect the surface, and the beauty and complexity evolve.

## Are You Undermining Your Commitment?

Commitment is a major and complex undertaking. It requires awareness of our motivations, needs, desires, and capabilities. In essence, it requires great maturity. Some people are able to embrace their relationship and all its commitments wholeheartedly. They never look back or question their personal choice. Their commitment is solid, a given.

For others, the requirements of commitment to another person and to a long-term relationship are less conscious or steadfast. Some people may not have considered all the ramifications of making such a choice, yet they find themselves in love and having made a commitment. Some people want to give up when times are tough. Others threaten to walk out to get their partner's attention. Some have worked hard to create a good relationship but get no cooperation from their partner; only at that point do they decide it is time to leave.

There are five basic behaviors that frequently undermine commitment:

- Making a commitment too soon in the relationship

- Abandoning oneself and consequently resenting one's partner

- Not living in alignment with one's values, goals, and priorities

- "Crying wolf" by threatening to leave or divorce

• Wanting to give up before one has tried everything possible to make the relationship successful

Let's take a look at each of these behaviors to see how it can chip away your commitment to your partner.

## Commitment Too Soon Creates a Weak Relationship

We have all heard stories of people who fall madly in love and decide to make a commitment to each other—to become engaged or get married—not long after their first date. In a number of these situations, the outcome is a long and happy relationship. Usually the two people are mature, know what they want in a mate, and are realistic about what it will take to create a relationship once they are committed.

Many other times, the outcome is not so positive. Sometimes a couple is too young. Jennifer and Jim are a case in point. Jennifer came to counseling while their divorce was being finalized. She wanted to avoid the pitfalls she and Jim had experienced in their young and short marriage. As Jennifer explained,

> Jim and I were just too young. We had no idea what marriage would require. All we knew was that we were head over heels for each other. At seventeen, you may think you are grown up, but there is so much to learn about life. Sadly to say, the marriage only lasted a year and a half. My parents were good about not saying, "I told you so."

As we spoke, Jennifer assessed that she and Jim had held a combination of Traditional and Merged styles when they got together. Over time, she wanted to develop her individual interests by going to school and working. Her need for personal development was threatening to Jim, who liked her being at home for him. He criticized her every action. At the time, Jennifer did not know quite what was wrong, but when she heard about Big Picture Partnering, she decided that this is the relationship style she will seek in her future. In the meantime, she's finishing her education and developing her personal interests, so that when the time is right, she will choose a mate more carefully.

Other times, a hasty commitment comes out of neediness. Carla remarked,

> I was on the rebound. I thought I had healed from my first marriage, which ended in a fairly amicable divorce after four years and no kids; however,

I should have taken more time to soul search. I just blamed Matt for our divorce and never stopped to look at my own shortcomings. As a result, I was pretty needy for affection and someone to lean on. These qualities didn't help either of my two marriages.

Very often people fall in love with a terrific person, but forget they are taking on an entire package of life experiences and extended family. Sometimes they may not understand the challenges that come with addictions or a history of dysfunction of any sort. Said Dan,

I thought she was the perfect person for me. She was gorgeous, fun loving, and ready to party. I'd never been married and was waiting for "Miss Right" to knock my socks off. Well, she did, all right. I just had no idea that everything about her past, as well as her behavior with me, should have been a red flag. She was a great gal, but she had troubles with alcohol, two kids from two different fathers, and was rarely employed for more than six months. She always wanted to go to the casino for entertainment and lost a lot of money. What was I thinking? I guess it was chemistry and a certain kind of love—but not the marrying kind of love!

Not all relationships can succeed. Sometimes the stressors are too great and the couple too ill-equipped. It takes solid maturity, an awareness of the long-term requirements of a relationship, education about the characteristics of a good mate, and a willingness to continuously work together to create a relationship and make it last.

## Abandoning Yourself Breeds Resentment

Internal abandonment is when your body is present, but your heart or mind is not fully involved in the moment—or in the relationship. Abandonment occurs when you are going through the motions, and so you say yes to things without really thinking or being committed to your choices.

Sometimes people abandon themselves and their partners for short periods of time. We all experience times like these when we are overly tired, distracted, or stressed by another area of life.

Harriet and Kammi are in their mid-forties and have been in a committed relationship for thirteen years. Sometimes Kammi "goes away" internally. As Harriet said,

I can always tell when Kammi is going through a stressful time at work. She comes home and she's like a robot. She'll come around after a few days, and then we talk about what's happening at work. Only then do I feel like I have her full attention once again.

Some people have a protective pattern they developed in childhood to shield themselves from being hurt. This pattern can cause one partner to go away internally. Gordon reports that his wife of thirty-two years would periodically go away internally, sometimes for weeks or even months. His wife went through the motions of daily life and had conversations with Gordon, yet she was not fully engaged in their relationship or in life:

Then one day, she'd just be "back." It was the most perplexing thing. We'd both know it. Later we learned that when someone or something shamed her, she withdrew. Shame was a constant part of her childhood and she had developed a protective mechanism to avoid the deep hurt it caused her. Learning about the Big Picture Partnering approach and the essentials help her stay present and talk out the hurt instead of withdrawing. It taught me how to be a better listener, and we now work through the issues together.

Some people don't take care of their physical or spiritual health. They may not exercise, or they may lack the vitality to have sex or engage in social pursuits. This physical withdrawal is another form of abandonment that has an impact on the individual as well as the partnership. Kim and Lee have been in a committed relationship for nineteen years, and recently Lee has exhibited this sort of physical distance. As Kim explained,

Lee and I had always enjoyed making love—and frequently. These days he's put on weight and seems vulnerable about getting older. I still find him attractive and loveable, but he's distracted and withdrawn. He's not even interested in going out for dinner or movies as often. We're still affectionate, but sex is very infrequent.

When you practice staying fully committed, you learn to be present in your relationship by taking time for yourself (to read, take a nap, go for a walk, see your friends, have a massage) so that you can feel refreshed. The two of you also learn to come together and go apart without having to internally withdraw, because you enjoy your individual activities and can count on regular times enjoying each other's company.

## Lacking Values and Priorities Undermines Your Relationship

While our society offers a myriad of exciting and wonderful options, many outside forces pose challenges to our personal relationships. In the modern world, we receive mixed messages about what to consider a priority, and we are faced with many temptations that guide us away from family life. While the reality of temptation and opportunities to stray is an issue that should be addressed in any intimate partnership, what I am referring to are the everyday socially acceptable temptations to stray from your core values. These include the temptations to

- spend money on bigger houses, cars, toys, vacations, or travel, and not pay attention to financial limits or future goals—because the economic system allows it;

- eat, drink, or exercise excessively;

- work excessively without considering the impact on your relationship and family in order to impress the boss and other colleagues;

- avoid too much involvement with your children, because you fear you might appear less professional to your colleagues or because you are not sure your children really want your involvement;

- prioritize house chores or home maintenance, rather than talking with or making love to your partner, because society leads us to believe that these things are more important;

- put friends or extended family above your partner.


All these socially acceptable, culturally approved behaviors tend to keep us from placing a priority on our relationship with our partner and our family. It is important to align our values and priorities, so that we can focus our energy on a committed partnership. Without this commitment couples flounder.

Cheryl's situation provides an example of how we create distractions that keep us from what's truly important. Thirty-four, a businesswoman and mother who has been married nine years, Cheryl had a habit of overspending that greatly interfered with her relationship. She admitted that she had a shopping addiction, that she would spend money to fill emotional requirements. When she was lonely or bored, she would buy toys for her young daughters when they did not need them. Her closet was filled with clothing that still had price tags on because she had too much to wear. She had purchased the items when she felt a little down or anxious. She had many ways of rationalizing her purchases and convinced herself that she and the kids deserved them, but she had lost the trust of her husband and felt ashamed. She overspent at department stores each month, racking up credit-card debt.

Cheryl had started counseling and had attended Spenders Anonymous meetings a few times but had not followed through on her commitment. When she and her husband, Jim, agreed to save for a bigger home for themselves and their two small children, Cheryl finally faced her priorities head on. Through individual counseling and then learning Big Picture skills with Jim, she reassessed her values and priorities and fully committed to her relationship and the goals she and Jim desired. This meant learning to not overspend. While resolving her spending addiction was very challenging for her, Cheryl sought ways to find internal happiness rather than distracting herself with external objects. She replaced time shopping after work with going to the gym with her friends while Jim picked the girls up from day care. She reconnected with her mother and talked about the origins of some of her anxieties, and these lessened. She and Jim talked about her loneliness and her need to reconnect with him and scheduled a date night at least once each week. They revitalized their affectionate behavior toward each other. Jim and Cheryl's mutual agreement about their financial priorities, and Cheryl's decision to face her internal priorities, helped her change her behavior—from spending to saving—so that it was aligned with the couple's desire for a new home. Today they have their new home, healthy preteen daughters, and a strong, committed Big Picture Partnership.

Martin's work environment challenged his relationship commitment. Married for thirty-seven years, he was a highly successful attorney, ran in a professional circle, and worked in an office in which men turned a blind eye to their colleagues' affairs. Family life was undermined by his expensive business trips, working late at the office, or having dinner with casual female friends. Alcohol was always a part of these gatherings.

Martin's wife, Mary, was committed to him and their two young children, yet he rationalized his extracurricular activities by pointing to the changes that marriage presented him. When they met, Mary had been athletic and active, but over the years, she had developed a chronic case of asthma that sometimes limited her activities. This change did not fit Martin's expectations of their relationship. He had not accepted or adjusted to fatherhood nor had he relinquished his bachelor way of life. He also worried that his professional life might suffer if he avoided the established carousing culture within his company. When he came to see me, Martin was terribly unhappy and filled with anxieties he hid from his wife. He knew something was awry about his entire life, and he feared losing both his family and his job if he did not take stock of what he truly wanted. He had no idea of how to do this on his own.

Martin faced some initial hard work individually in order to align his life with his core values. To feel more grounded at home, he stopped fighting with Mary and started the Big Picture Partnering Steps 1 and 2 by increasing the positives and talking regularly. Then he reevaluated his life and privately renewed his commitment to their relationship while he sorted out his confusion. This commitment helped him refocus his life at home and at work. After much soul searching, Martin decided to reorganize his work life to reflect values he thought he wanted to follow at this stage of his life. He realized that he had spent enough years having the freedom and fun of a bachelor. He had chosen to marry, have children, and enter into family life. Now he wanted to learn how to fully participate in and enjoy this choice. He was already very successful in his career. Enlisting the support of his businessman father, his wife, and a few close friends, Martin sought feedback on how to make the change he needed within his current company. He went over his boss's head and was able to work under a new supervisor with more stable values. As Martin and Mary continued to talk and strengthen their partnering commitment, Martin discovered things to do with his free time and recommitted time to his family. While he had always been a man with seemingly inexhaustible energy, once he aligned his values with his day-to-day life, Martin found that the lack of anxiety and guilt resulted in even more energy. He channeled this energy into the things he wanted now and in his future. He grew to appreciate more deeply what he had built in his life, and he found healthier ways of letting off steam and playing. He and Mary partnered on creating a new relationship, one that supported their individuals needs and also reflected their more mature relationship.

In both of these situations, a number of options presented themselves, and various paths could have been taken. While making skillful choices can be confusing, when we reflect on our priorities and realign our life choices to reflect the core commitments we embrace, we can make decisions that create inner peace and are in sync with our Big Picture Partnership.

While extended family, friends, bosses, and coworkers may challenge your decisions—because it may mean less time at the golf course, the shopping mall, the office, family events, or social functions—those who truly care about you will respect, even admire and support, that you are striving to reflect your mutual values and strengthen your relationship. If they truly care about you, they will work to find ways to be with you that align with your time and availability.

## Threatening to Leave or Divorce Is Harmful

Another way of abandoning a relationship is to create instability by threatening to leave or divorce. Even when separation or divorce is not truly intended, such threats are ominous and loom over a relationship. They typically contain an element of the partner's thoughts, even when he or she claims it was "just a joke." Usually such threats are meant to get a rise out of the partner and come from the Critical Parent or Wounded Child state.

Unless you stay very adult, it is easy to slip into a childlike demand for attention or parental criticism. For example, "Well! I guess you don't really love me or you'd stay home and we'd go out tonight!" may come from your Wounded Child if you are feeling neglected. A Critical Parent might lash out and say, "This is never going to work! You simply don't ever listen to my needs, even the little ones like keeping the house clean. I've had it!"

We know that children will seek attention through negative behaviors if attention is not freely given when they are behaving positively. Even as adults, we are prone to do the same when we are not in our solid Adult Self. When faced with lack of attention, perceived lack of attention, or when you have other unmet needs, you can present your unhappiness in a way that will be more effective; in a way that will not threaten your partner or your entire relationship.

---

**TIP:** A basic rule of commitment is, never threaten to leave, never threaten divorce, unless you truly mean it. Then presenting your need should be done in an adult way—seriously, respectfully, with care for your partner's potentially angry, defensive, or sad response.

---

Here are examples of individuals who threatened their spouse in order to get their attention and to provoke a change of behavior or, failing that, a fight that might indicate their spouse's love. Instead, their tactic backfired and got them just what they did not want. Their partner became more withdrawn.

Anna and John have been married for six years. She is in her early thirties, and he is pushing forty. Anna wanted a bigger home and to start a family. John appeared content with their very busy life of work and socializing with a group of friends. He is a strong, silent type; Anna craves more verbal and emotional connection. She's discontent with their Roommate Style:

After a while I just didn't know how to reach John. He'd simply mumble or put me off when I wanted to talk about a new house or trying to get pregnant. He is a master at avoiding. Instead of creating conflict, he tried to humor me. But I was getting furious and started to say things like, "Maybe you never wanted kids and I do. Maybe this marriage won't work after all. You lied to me about having a family." I started to yell at him frequently, and he withdrew. I really didn't want to end our marriage. His silence still bugs me, but I love so many other things about him. I just want him to talk to me. I learned through Big Picture Partnering how damaging these threats can be. We finally got help and learned to talk more openly. And I discovered through our talks how afraid he was that I would really leave.

Another example of "crying wolf" threatening their relationship is Henry and Sarah. Henry is an active guy. Becoming a father with family obligations was challenging for him. He felt Sarah didn't divide her time well between him and their one-year-old. Henry described that instead of talking to her, he'd tell Sarah,

Maybe I'm just not cut out for parenthood. We never go out anymore. You seem totally content with whatever Danny needs—and I get frustrated. Maybe we're not meant to be together.

Sarah ended up sad and frustrated with Henry's summation of their marriage. To protect herself she withdrew even further and gave even more attention to their child. In her mind, she began to prepare for the possibility that Henry might leave someday. As a result, Henry became more frustrated with her withdrawal and passivity in the relationship until it all came to a head and the truth about their feelings came out in an initial session in my office. As Henry related,

Here I thought I was trying to tell her I wanted more time with her—not to take away from our child, whom I love—but to let her know I loved lots of the things we used to do, and the joy she brings me when we are doing more things together. I guess I chose a pretty lousy way of expressing it. Sarah finally told me she was even thinking about where she and Danny could live, how she'd manage financially, while at the same time she was hoping I'd wake up to what a good thing we had going. That's when we finally got some help to communicate better. I could have lost Sarah and Danny if I had kept saying those threatening things—when all I wanted was to be closer again.

Often when partners threaten to walk out of a relationship, or to divorce, they are "crying wolf." They have thought about ending the relationship in passing, perhaps, but their intention in airing this thought is to get closer to their partner or simply to elicit a reaction or attention from their mate. On the other hand, it could mean that they have seriously thought about ending the relationship. No matter your intention, telling your partner that you want to leave the relationship damages trust. Even if intellectually they know you don't really mean it, it will set up a negative pattern between you—getting you exactly what you don't want.

### Wanting to Give up Before You've Tried Everything Possible

When couples claim that they want to break up, I ask them to reconsider. They need to think about any regrets they might have if they do not try to sort out the problems in their relationship. Breaking up and divorce have long-lasting consequences for both the adults and the children involved.

Seeking help at this point means attending relationship therapy or participating in a marriage education course. It means learning new skills, looking at the issues, and arriving at potential new solutions. This is important for two reasons: 1) As we get older, we cannot help but accumulate more regrets, and 2) regrets and feelings of failure are hard on the heart. For the sake of your heart and your future well-being, make sure you know for certain that you have done all you can to make the relationship work.

The second reason to get help for your relationship is for your children's sake. As adults, you and your partner will survive and rebuild your lives. Your children, no matter what their ages, will be affected by your threatening their stability and breaking up their home. While many children adjust to these changes that come with divorce, they will always live with the psychological and emotional ramifications of their parents breaking apart. They are also likely to experience the inconsistency, instability, and negative economics of divorce, no matter how well they are parented by one or both of you.

## One Day at a Time

One study shows that when married couples are unhappy but stay together even though they don't get outside help, 86 percent report greatly increased happiness and satisfaction five years later. The experts speculate that much of a couple's dissatisfaction may be due to circumstances—such as job stress, child rearing, health problems, care of elderly parents, disability, etc. If they stay together, such circumstances pass with time. When couples survive difficult times and, additionally, seek support and learn to partner during those times, they can thrive.

I always advise couples going through stressful situations to commit to working on their relationship on a daily basis—one day at a time. Every morning, acknowledge your commitment by saying to yourself, "I am willing to do my part in partnering today." When your circumstances are difficult, in order to weather the daily ups and downs, use your sense of willingness to help you build the emotional muscles and stamina to stay in the relationship and keep moving forward. Of course, you should seek support and help. Moreover, if you need a break, take a few hours off just for yourself. Offer your partner time off as well.

## If You Are Considering Leaving Your Partner

Sometimes a breakup or divorce is unavoidable. If a couple must break up or divorce, it is important that the partners try to separate without threats or anger. As doing so can be extremely difficult in some cases, many couples seek professional help to get through this difficult process. Again, I always advise couples who are on the brink of separation to make absolutely certain that dissolving their partnership is what they want to do. If they discuss their potential breakup with a psychologist, marriage counselor, or mediator and still decide to end their relationship, at least they will have a better understanding of "why" and less opportunity for regrets and bitterness down the road.

There are many challenges, circumstances, and phases in a long-term relationship. Some are more difficult and some more joyful than others. If we love our partner in the active way that M. Scott Peck describes, if in our calmer moments we truly want to be in a relationship, if we are mature enough to know that the day-to-day is not always easy, then commitment to the relationship—along with perseverance, creativity, and humor—can see us through the challenging times.

## Children and Divorce

It is not uncommon in stressful marriages for the kids to weigh in on whether parents should stay together or divorce. **DO NOT** give your children this power. Keep them out of the middle. This is your adult relationship and you need to deal with it, whether you stay together or separate. It is harmful to children when they take sides. It is harmful to children to see the two of you act in ways they don't respect—you are their role models—even if they see you disagree and divorce. If they see you acting as adults and treating each other, as well as them, respectfully, you will all be better off.

You are the adults, and they need to be the children. What is important is learning to communicate appropriately with your children about times of stress that may feel threatening to them. It is best if you can partner on how and what to communicate to your kids. If you cannot partner, then you be the stable, healthy, appropriately adult parent in your communications. These communications include the following:

- Reassure your children that you love them and will always take care of them.

- NEVER confide in your children. This is a burden they are too young to manage. Talk to your healthy friends and a therapist.

- Let them know that adults do have problems and tell them the truth about what you are doing. For example: "Yes, your daddy and I are having problems. He's very mad at me and sometimes I don't speak kindly to him. Even adults need to practice healthy communication. Even adults need to learn better ways of talking to each other so they don't hurt each other."

- Then tell them more truth. "We are going to counseling to learn how to treat each other better." Or, "We are going to live in two separate houses for a while to see if we can learn to be nicer to each other." Either way, say, "This is our adult problem. We still love you and your job is to be the kid. We will always love you and take care of you."

- Never mention divorce unless you have finalized that decision. Kids know it is a possibility. What they don't know is if you are working on your relationship. Unless you tell them, they will jump to conclusions.

- Tell your children you are going to take five minutes every other day to talk with them about how they are feeling. Do this with each child individually, giving each child an opportunity to open up and have you just listen. You can reassure and clarify what is going on if you hear their fear or their misunderstanding.

Good luck. Make sure to get the help you need, especially if you have children and you are separating or headed for divorce. You and your mate will need partnering skills for many years to come because they are always your children.

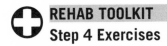

**REHAB TOOLKIT**
## Step 4 Exercises

### *Affirming Your Sense of Commitment*

This week, I'd like each of you, on your own, to deepen your commitment. Say the following affirmations out loud to yourself each day:

- I am willing to continuously choose our relationship. I'm willing to work at our relationship, even when I am tired or the going gets tough.

- I choose to be creative in our relationship. I choose to learn new ways of doing things if the old ways are not working.

- I am committed to our relationship because I value it. I know that we can make it more and more solid and exciting if we do it together.

- I am willing to protect our relationship through my words and actions. I will work to surround our relationship with healthy people and participate in healthy activities.

How do these affirmations resonate inside you? If you like, rewrite them in your own words. You might also add other affirmations as well.

Write them out and put them on the bathroom mirror or on your dashboard to remind you of your commitment to your relationship.

As you begin to say these affirmations every day, notice any changes in your behavior, attitudes, willingness, or feelings of being present or engaged in your relationship.

## Are You Undermining Your Commitment to Your Relationship?

Take some time to reflect on what you learned in this chapter about the subtle ways you may inadvertently or indirectly abandon your relationship. Abandonment, even subtle, can potentially undermine your commitment. Ask yourself the following questions to clarify any of the ways you may be indirectly abandoning your partner. You may think of other examples. Write the following questions and your answers in your notebook:

- In what ways do I keep one foot in and, at the same time, keep one foot out of my relationship?

- Am I putting other activities (chores, time with my friends, hobbies) before time with my partner?

- Do I tend to tune out and not really listen when I come home from a long day?

- Does my commitment to work overshadow my commitment to my partner and family?

- When I am tired, excited, or frustrated, do I overspend, drink too much, or stay out later than I promised?

- Am I telling my partner what I really think or avoiding the truth because I'm afraid of hurt or angry feelings, or am I stuffing it under the rug because I feel a little lazy and hope my concerns will go away?

- If I'm not talking about a concern I have in our relationship, am I gradually withdrawing affection? Am I too tired for sex or disinterested in time together?

- Am I hanging out with people who undermine long-term relationships and commitment?

Spend some time with these questions. They are tough. They are about the ways we erode confidence in and commitment to our relationships.

Abandoning ourselves—by not taking care of ourselves—is another way we commonly abandon our partnerships. We get worn out, stressed out. We come home too tired, too harried, too distracted to have anything to offer our most important relationship. Consider the following statement: "If I don't fully take care of me, I have abandoned me."

In what ways does this statement apply to you? How has it affected your life, your partner, and your relationship?

## Protection from Outside Pressures

Ask yourself if your relationship is experiencing any outside distractions or pressures. Make a list of even small pressures or distractions you or your partner might be feeling. What would be the consequences of removing these distractions and pressures? Bring these reflections to your conversation with your partner.

## Sharing with Your Partner

When the two of you are ready, later this week, come together and share what you are noticing about your commitment. Take turns listening to each other.

## Chapter 7

# STEP 5:

## Address Any Issue Together— Whether It's Yours, Mine, or Ours

In the initial steps of this program you have focused on rebuilding your foundation: calming things down and increasing positive interactions (Step 1), listening to each other again (Step 2), learning to stay Adult (Step 3), and staying committed no matter what is going on between you (Step 4). Continuing to integrate each of these foundational steps will strengthen your connection. Keeping your connection strong is necessary as you move forward—learning a new perspective and new ways to constructively work through your problems together. In this chapter, you will learn **Big Picture Step 5: Address Any Issue Together—Whether It's Yours, Mine, or Ours**. Adding this step to your toolkit will stretch you beyond your personal limits to include consideration and care for another—your partner. In Big Picture Partnering, you are inclusive and expansive of your partner, knowing your partner will do the same for you. You are in this together.

In addition, you are both attending to and inclusive of the entire Partnership Universe. This Universe includes everything: your world, my world, our mutual world, your commitments and agreements, your words and activities, your joys and sorrows, your dreams and desires, and so on. In this chapter, you will reflect on becoming more inclusive and openhearted—fully nurturing each other and your partnership. When you develop a heartfelt, inclusive approach it opens the way for you to experience vibrancy and joy in your lives.

On a day-to-day level, the communications and actions that accompany Step 5 reflect your willingness to consider all needs or requests equally and to address them together as partners—even if they are not your needs, even when they are not important to you.

## Addressing Any Problem in Your Relationship Together

One of the most difficult things in any relationship is to acknowledge that our partner may experience aspects of our relationship differently than we do. Things that make us feel content, happy, or even neutral may be bothersome or downright annoying to our partner. For example, the amount of clutter, amount of time spent on the telephone, rising early or going to bed late are common differences that many partners face. What may seem benign to one of you may drive the other "crazy" like the proverbial toilet seat; what causes you no pain or sadness may be painful to your partner. For example, a harsh tone that you use in business may remind him or her of a father's abusive language when your partner was young. As you strengthen your partnership, you are expanding your awareness that what affects one of you affects both of you. As partners, you become responsible for creating a nurturing environment and addressing any issues that come up for one or the other or both of you. You do this because you generously and openheartedly want your partnership and each other to flourish; your partner wants the same.

---

**TIP:** In Big Picture Partnering, anything that is a problem, issue, or complaint for one person is automatically an issue for the partnership, because you agree to meet all three categories of needs—yours, mine, or ours together. When you do this, both the individuals and the partnership can flourish.

---

Addressing issues in any relationship is more difficult when one person is content and the other sees a problem. Jane and Anna's relationship is a case in point.

Jane and Anna have intermittent eruptions in their relationship, partly because Anna is more outgoing, while Jane is more contained. Anna reverts to childlike acting out of her anger to get attention, while Jane becomes overly calm and unresponsive. Jane thinks the relationship would be just fine if Anna would only stop acting out. When questioned, Anna knows she wants Jane's undivided attention a little more often. She feels that communication takes place only when Jane wants it to happen.

Then there are Brian and Suzanne. Brian also feels his relationship is just fine, but Suzanne admits to feeling frustrated and throwing tantrums to get Brian to talk to her about things she feels are important. She is dissatisfied with the frequency of sex. She is concerned about whether they should buy a bigger house and whether they're going to have children—she wants them; Brian is ambivalent. She also wants Brian to be more emotionally responsive and to give her undivided attention at times. Brian dismisses Suzanne's pleas for discussion to resolve these issues. He thinks their relationship is pretty good just the way it is. He's not sure he wants children, and he feels that Suzanne would need to calm down in order for him to ever consider having children with her.

To get to the root of what each of these couples calls a stalemate, we decided to use a scale to explore the similarities and differences in satisfaction level and the degrees to which each partner felt individual needs were being met. Both Jane and Brian said their satisfaction level was at 7 or 8 on a scale of from 1 to 10. Each of them was getting 70 to 80 percent of their needs met. That's pretty high.

On the other hand, Jane's partner Anna and Brian's partner Suzanne reported a satisfaction level of 4 to 5 on the ten-point scale, in comparison to their partner's rating of 7 or 8. This is quite a difference in perception of satisfaction and needs. No wonder both couples had a stalemate.

This difference in contentment regarding one or many aspects in a relationship is not uncommon. Yet many couples continue with the status quo even when one person is not fully happy. At these times, the more contented person in the relationship wields power when he or she dismisses the partner's unhappiness or concerns. When this power is paired with denial of, or lack of empathy for, a mate's pain or a dismissal of a partner's needs as unnecessary or frivolous, then unconscious power becomes uncaring. In any relationship, if something affects you adversely, it is eventually going to affect your partner. To safeguard against a lack of mutual happiness or contentment, Big Picture Partnering makes lack of contentment a partnering issue. Jane and Brian can deny or ignore that there is a problem between them and their partners. On the other hand, they are both experiencing the unhappy consequences of their mate's dissatisfaction. Both Anna and Suzanne admit to acting out their dissatisfaction regularly, either by picking fights, crying, complaining, or criticizing their mate.

---

**TIP:** Two people in a relationship typically move in life at different "speeds." One may change quickly; one may like things the way they are and change slowly, if at all. You can only go as fast as the slowest person in the relationship. The slowest person, therefore, has more power. In choosing to partner, you choose to come partway toward each other. You each take responsibility for change.

---

Sometimes partners will deny there is a problem in the relationship because they feel helpless to respond to the other person's needs, or they don't know how both of them could have their needs met at the same time. This might apply to Brian and Suzanne's situation, in which one definitely wants a child and the other is ambivalent. Rather than avoiding communication about difficult or heated topics, the Big Picture approach—using all 10 Steps—can provide safe ways to talk through and ultimately resolve difficult issues. I have seen many partners gracefully work through their seemingly irresolvable issues in that way. If the issues are too big to deal with on your own, agree as partners to get help from a trained pastor, marriage educator, mentor, or therapist.

Let's explore some other thoughts that contribute to being inclusive— learning to expand your awareness and responsiveness to include not only you, but also your partner and the our world you share. The entirety of the Big Picture Universe is your partnership. Practicing Step 5 will assist you in developing an expansive mind and heart that helps you stay inclusive—aware and open to this vibrant Relationship Universe the two of you are creating together.

Let's explore this large concept of inclusiveness and reflect on some additional features that are a part of practicing this essential step. These include

- reminding yourselves that partnering is a joint effort;

- pulling your weight in the partnership, no matter what your partner is doing;

- making and keeping clear agreements with each other.

## Partnering Is a Joint Effort

In Big Picture Partnering, the two of you are teammates, even when you are in disagreement. You are willing to work toward perceiving your partner as your teammate, not your adversary. You remember that your individuality and needs are safeguarded in the 10 Steps of the Big Picture. Therefore, you can always consider both your personal needs and those of your relationship without being afraid that you will lose out.

When balancing individual and partnership needs, some people are too rigidly individualistic and others are wishy-washy, giving in too easily and always wanting to be liked, loved, or perceived as good or wanted. Sometimes we say yes or no too quickly and don't benefit from adding another point of view to the discussion. We also live in a world riddled with subtle everyday polarization. It is a world of us versus them. Often we feel that there won't be enough to go around—enough pieces of the pie, enough money, enough love, enough time, enough recognition, enough abundance to fulfill and sustain all aspects of our lives. So we think that we are involved in a battle, forgetting the bonds that tie us together as human beings.

It takes two mature people to stay out of the tug-of-war game that is so prevalent in relationships.

It may take more time to listen carefully to each other and come to an agreement that considers both parties and meets both of your needs. However, taking time is certainly better than taking an adversarial stance.

To help you keep an inclusive, openhearted attitude, especially in times of stress, surround yourself with friends and relationships that are also inclusive. Nourish each other with high positive interactions (Step 1). Consistently talk and listen to each other (Step 2). Build the muscles of a healthy Adult Self and do something nice for yourself (Step 3). Remain fully committed to each other (Step 4). Then, when you become aware of a difference between you and your partner, treating each other as teammates rather than as enemies, as friends rather than as foes, will be easier. You will be able to listen for understanding and work toward resolution from a more inclusive and loving perspective.

## Pull Your Weight into the Partnership, No Matter What Your Partner Is Doing

When learning new ways to improve a relationship, it is helpful if both partners implement the necessary changes all of the time. However, from time to time we all succumb to behaviors that thwart change and prevent partnering. Let me describe a few of these behaviors, and see if you recognize them in yourselves.

I'm sure you have heard the old phrase, "tit for tat." Many couples fall into this trap of retaliating for an alleged wrongdoing, of judging the other person's behavior before considering their own, of blaming their mate and waiting for them to change. The rationale in tit for tat is that, "They really are to blame, so I won't do anything to improve the situation until they do." Typically, this leads to a stalemate, because both parties are looking for the other person to change first.

Another phrase you will recognize is, "We are only human." When we say this, the usual implication is that we know we didn't follow through on a promise or resolution, but we can't really do anything about it; after all, "We're only human." We're aware that we let others or ourselves down, but we use the excuse that everyone makes mistakes—and we fail to consider what we might do next time to prevent making the same blunder.

For some couples, such attitudes and behaviors are especially common in times of stress, transition, or learning new ways to behave. For some couples, they are daily bad habits.

As you begin practicing Big Picture Partnering, be prepared for those times when you will fall off the wagon. One of you is going to have a bad day or a tough week. Under stress, someone is going to forget to experiment with the new behaviors and approaches to partnering. It is a given. No matter how hard we try to be perfect, it is just not possible.

Kathlyn and Gay Hendricks, fellow marriage educators and authors of *Conscious Loving: The Journey to Co-Commitment*, describe the best remedy for such common relationship pitfalls. The Hendricks assign each person in the relationship 100-percent responsibility for doing his or her part. This is not a 50-50 relationship, it is a 200-percent interaction.

If we refer back to the parent/adult/child model, 100-percent responsibility means staying adult even when your partner is letting the Wounded Child run amok. It means staying adult when your partner is in the Critical Parent Self, blaming you for something you may or may not have done. You have full responsibility for applying the 10 Steps of Big Picture Partnering to your relationship all of the time, even when your partner isn't.

## Becoming Impeccable

Another way of thinking about pulling your weight in Big Picture Partnering is continuing to do your part, no matter what anyone else is doing. I call this *impeccable behavior*. Impeccable behavior implies that you do what is correct in any given situation, even if you don't want to or if the going gets tough. It means putting the 10 Steps of the partnership first—keeping the Big Picture in mind and minimizing day-to-day bad habits. This perspective is even more important to remember when you are not in a good mood, you have had a bad day, or you and your partner are working through some difficult issues or differences. If your partner is under stress, you might sometimes be alone in your practice of these essentials for a short while. Try to remain consistent, impeccable, inclusive, and openhearted. Usually your partner will rejoin you.

---

**TIP:** If you find that your partner withdraws from partnering for a long time, stay with the practice as much as you can. If needed, seek outside help to get to the bottom of the issues preventing you both from acting on your commitment to Big Picture Partnering and the 10 Steps. Get to the bottom of the issues on your own or together—with help.

---

## Make and Keep Clear Agreements with Each Other

This principle states that you are a responsible, mature individual. Therefore, you willingly do what you agree to do within the period you said you would do it. It implies that you only make agreements that are true to your Big Picture Partnership and yourself and that you are including your partner in your thoughts, agreements, and actions. You are saying, "I realize I have an impact on you, and I'm going to follow through on what I agreed to do. And if I cannot follow through for some reason, I'll let you know and we will figure out another away to accomplish the task." It doesn't matter how big or small the agreement is.

In any relationship, when you follow through on your agreements, you build trust. Your friends, family, coworkers, and partner learn to count on you. Some people call this walking your talk. Typically, people who make clear agreements and act on them do so in every facet of their lives. Let's look at how Frank and Jen laid the foundation for establishing their Big Picture Partnering Style agreements early on in their relationship.

When they first met, Frank said he would call Jen early in the following week to ask her out—and he did just that. In the early stages of their courtship, he'd call every Monday morning to ask Jen about her plans for that Friday or Saturday night. They would make a date, and he always showed up on time. Gradually, Frank started asking Jen if she would also like to get together on Tuesday evenings for dinner. This went on for a few weeks until he began to call just to talk once or twice during the week. Jen let him take the lead to see how dependable Frank would be. Eventually they agreed that they should share the calling and the initiating of plans, but they could count on Tuesday and one weekend night as they grew to know each other better.

From this early courtship behavior, Jen learned to trust that Frank would do what he agreed to do. She realized he was a man of his word, carefully building her confidence and trust in the sincerity of his interest. He discovered he could trust her responsiveness to his invitations and gradually to making larger decisions together. They have been married for eighteen years now, and Frank is always accountable and clear in his agreements with Jen. They have had their challenges over the years, but accountability is not one of them.

Some people have difficulty living up to their agreements. They confuse their partners, friends, and associates by saying yes and then not following through on what they agreed to do. In any relationship, especially an intimate one, such lack of accountability always leads to distrust, anger, and frustration on the part of the mate, and shame, anger, and sometimes denial or avoidance on the part of the person who makes unclear agreements or fails to follow through. I am thinking about David, who, in the early stages of our couples coaching, frequently stated his intentions to engage in Big Picture Partnering with his wife, Eileen. He made such statements with regard to mundane issues—such as sharing the responsibility for household chores—as well as deeper ones—such as attending to Eileen's need for affection and acknowledging the positive things she contributed to their marriage.

Although Eileen could trust David to follow through on his agreement to care for their son when he said he would, she could not count on him to do the household chores or to give her a hug or otherwise express affection or appreciation. David reverted to the Roommate Style of relating and unilaterally decided when he would or would not give affection. He would forget to do the chores or he would become too overwhelmed. Eileen could not count on what he said he would do, which led to deep and ongoing strife. This couple could not fully engage in Big Picture Partnering because David consistently failed to act on many of his agreements.

In addition to being honest about what you will and won't agree to in your relationship, each of you can become skilled at indicating a need for more time to reflect on what you are willing to agree to in any situation. For example,

- Your partner may learn to say, "I need to think about it," and "I will get back to you later this week." And he will follow through later that week.

- You will learn to say, "I don't have time to do that this week, but how about next Wednesday?" And you will follow through next Wednesday.

- You may both learn to indicate, "I never thought about that. Let me think it over, and then I'd be happy to tell you my thoughts either over dinner tomorrow night or at our weekly family meeting next Sunday." And then you will both follow through at those times. You will both feel good because you have been inclusive, openhearted Big Picture Partners!

## A Word about Sabotage

As you proceed through the exercises in the coming chapters you will be asked to reflect on ways you *sabotage* your progress. In a dictionary, the original meaning of sabotage refers to "the destruction of property." Here, I am referring to the potential to destroy or hinder progress toward your desire to become a Big Picture Partner.

Ways in which we sabotage ourselves may be large or small. Some examples that fit this program may include

- withholding a compliment when I know it would please my partner;

- "forgetting" an agreement with my partner;

- eating or drinking too much so I have no energy for sex;

- oversleeping when the morning is my best time to read the chapters in this book and reflect on the exercises;

- trying to convince my partner to watch TV instead of talking together about the exercises at the end of each chapter;

- avoiding scheduling regular talking time on a consistent basis;

- cleaning the house instead of making time for a date night.

### ✚ REHAB TOOLKIT
### How Do I Sabotage My Relationship?

Reflect for a minute on the typical ways you avoid, hinder, or impair your progress toward general goals in your life. Then think about any ways in which you have been sabotaging or hindering your own progress or your partner's progress during the past few weeks. Make a list of all the ways you sabotage your relationship's success. Before you begin the exercises at the end of this chapter, state your intention to not sabotage—both in your notebook and aloud during a regular talking time with your partner.

Now that you have completed this chapter, individually and together, reflect on your readiness to use *Step 5:* Address Any Issue Together—Whether It's Yours, Mine, or Ours, and the perspective of inclusiveness and openheartedness that comprises true compassion. In the following exercises, you will explore the attitudes and behaviors that characterize this essential step, such as reminding yourselves that partnering is a joint effort, pulling your weight in the partnership no matter what your partner is doing, and making and keeping clear agreements with each other.

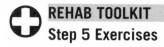

## REHAB TOOLKIT
### Step 5 Exercises

### *Four Questions*

Spend some time individually reflecting on your readiness to address any issue—be it yours, mine, or ours—and to be openhearted and inclusive. Write in your notebook about ways you find the concepts discussed in this chapter to be easy and/or challenging. In your notebook, also explore the following four questions:

1. Am I willing and committed to become fully inclusive of our entire Big Picture Universe? Am I openhearted to everything that is yours, mine, and ours—the good stuff and the tough stuff (differences, issues, etc.)? Am I willing to address any issue in our relationship together, remind myself that partnering is a joint effort, pull my weight no matter what my partner is doing, and make and keep clear agreements?
2. What are four specific, concrete steps I can take this week to live according to this commitment?
3. How might I sabotage or get in the way of this commitment? Give examples here.
4. What support would I like from my partner in order to keep my commitment?

### *Sharing Your Readiness*

Share your reflections from the four questions with your partner during your regular talking time. Take turns deciding your answers to the four questions. One of you should simply ask the question and listen to the answer. You are to witness only—no response is allowed. Take turns doing this for each other.

Now, using your notebook, explore the following four questions about making clear agreements and acting on them.

1. Am I willing and committed to address any concern or need—my own or my partner's—as a partnership concern?
2. What are four specific things I can do to consider my partner's concerns more fully? What are four things I can do to express my concerns more openly?
3. How might I sabotage, or get in the way of perceiving, both our needs as partnership needs?
4. What support do I need from my partner to help me do all of these things?

**Chapter 8**

# STEP 6:

## Understand How You Manage Conflict

You've probably noticed as you practice Steps 1–5 of this approach that improving your relationship requires change in your perspective and attitude, your behaviors and communications. You've probably also noticed that communication includes not only *what* you say but also *how* you speak and the *intention* behind your interaction. **Big Picture Step 6: Understand How You Manage Conflict** will help you assess your conflict style. Clarifying how you respond to differences and disagreements will help you become less reactive, less stuck on past behaviors, as you integrate all 10 Steps and become creative problem solvers together.

### Common Communication Wisdom

Even before the research was completed on relationship longevity and communication styles in long-term couples, much was known about basic, good communication. If you are Big Picture Partners, this common wisdom is fundamental. You are probably already using most of these guidelines. If not, refresh yourself with the following to increase your awareness and skill.

## Use "I" Messages When Speaking

"I" messages tell of your inner experience. For example, "I want to please you right now, but the kids need help with their homework. I'd like us both to help them, and then we can relax once they are in bed. Would that work for you?" Let your partner tell you his or her inner experience and be willing to listen to it.

## Don't "Mind Read"

Mind reading is trying to figure out, or assuming that you already know, what your partner is thinking or feeling. It is telling your partner what he or she is thinking and feeling rather than listening to what that person has to say. Also, don't expect your partner to be able to read your mind.

## Speak for Yourself

In adult interactions, it is best if each person speaks for himself or herself. It helps if you don't prejudge your partner's thoughts or feelings. Each of you has a separate inner experience, and each experience is valid. One does not negate the other. It is easier for your partner to listen to you if you "speak for yourself," plus, your partner is more willing to open up and talk to you if he or she feels safe and listened to.

## Listen Actively

When you are in the listener role, show that you are interested and tracking what your partner is saying through eye contact, facial expression, and even sounds ("hmmm" or "oh" or other appropriate vocal gestures).

## Be Respectful

Think of how you would communicate if you did so with grace and dignity. You would never swear at, berate, or belittle your partner. You wouldn't interrupt. You would definitely not blame, shame, or criticize. You wouldn't raise your voice. Neither would you tease inappropriately, use sarcasm, or do anything that had a hurtful intent.

Instead, you would choose your words carefully when delivering thoughts that might cause pain, concern, or anger. I don't mean you would mince your words or treat another adult like a child who can't handle feedback or critique. Rather, you would communicate with the intention to achieve understanding versus an intention to harm or drive the other person away.

# More Than Words

In Chapter 3, we discussed the importance of Dr. Gottman's 5-to-1 ratio of positive interactions. Gottman's research findings on marital success or divorce also include factors that are less about *what you say* and more about *how you interact* and *your positive or negative intent*. For example, Gottman's predictors of marital success and happiness include the following.

## High Levels of Friendship, Respect, Affection, and Humor

This is defined as liking each other, being each other's best friend, doing things together, showing interest, supporting each other's goals and aspirations, having fun and laughing together, and being Number One in each other's eyes.

## Successful Bids for Attention

For example, the wife says, "Hey, listen to this!" and her husband keeps watching TV and ignores her. He's turning away her bid for attention. However, if he lifts his head and looks at her saying, "Huh?" he's turning toward her. If he actually listens to what she says or starts a conversation, that's a real connection! In successful relationships, couples turn toward each other 86 percent of the time while divorcing couples turn toward each other a mere 33 percent of the time.

## Soft Starts

Disagreements are started softly, without criticism, blame, or a harsh tone.

## Husband Accepts Influence from Wife

In successful relationships, the husband listens to his wife's advice and will consider changing his behavior based on her observations. Of course, this goes both ways, but women have more experience with accepting influence from their partners. Gottman notes it is important for men to do the same.

## Awareness of Each Other's Likes, Needs, Dislikes, and Inner Life

Partners notice each other's preferences; they ask questions; they listen; they care.

The predictors of divorce in Gottman's research include harsh starts of arguments, attacking character traits instead of the problem, name-calling, eye-rolling, contempt, sarcasm, defensiveness, withdrawal, silence, and failing to accept your partners attempts to apologize, ease the tension, or reconnect.

## ✚ REHAB TOOLKIT:
## How Do I Contribute to Our Success?

The previous lists highlight the basic ways you can open—or slam shut—the door to connecting with your partner. The ways we interact are not complicated, but they are powerful. Stop and reflect for a moment. Write in your notebook. Ask yourself, "How do I contribute to our interactions in both positive and negative ways? How do I behave and talk in ways that promote safety, friendship, and openness between us? In what ways do I threaten the longevity and success of our relationship?" Be specific. Refer back to these lists and make a thorough list of your negative behaviors and verbalizations. Own up to them and ask yourself, "What is my intention when I do this negative behavior or say something hurtful to my partner?" (For example, you might lash out so he or she will stop nagging you to follow through on the household chores you said you would do. What else could you do instead?) Ask yourself if you are willing to learn another way of getting your needs met as you continue working through this program.

Reminding yourself about the basic rules of communication in the lists above should be a given in your relationship. If you've forgotten to use them, make an agreement with yourself to start now.

---

Incorporating these basic rules of communication may not be enough to resolve the unresolved issues in your relationship—but it is a start! In the next section, you will learn about the different ways that couples approach disagreements and see how some couples are more effective in resolving their conflicts than others. Then we will discuss how you can effectively partner in successfully resolving your own conflicts so you can mutually work toward creative solutions together.

## Different Approaches to Conflict and What Works

Fighting, arguing, and disagreeing (some people call any type of disagreement a fight, even silence or withdrawing) are normal in any relationship. It's not problematic to disagree or argue as long as you keep many more positive interactions and feelings flowing, as you learned in *Step 1*: Increase the Positive Between You. Long-term, ongoing, out-and-out fighting in which nothing is resolved or couples make threats is very damaging to any relationship. The same is true of relationships in which there is a lack of conflict and disagreements are pushed under the rug—to be tripped over later. The research on long-term couples is conclusive about two aspects of conflict, disagreement, and fighting:

- *Couples need safe and mutual ground rules for disagreements or fights.* Such rules allow them to share their different points of view and be listened to and understood by their partner, even if their partner doesn't share the same point of view.

- *Coming to resolution creates greater contentment and longevity.* Feeling competent in resolving differences, disagreements, or fights strengthens a relationship, be it agreeing to take turns ("I'll have sex your way today, and you do it my way next week; I'll visit your relatives this month, and you visit my relatives at the holiday."), agreeing to disagree ("I see you can't stand these friends of mine, so I'll see them on my own, and neither of us will expect you to ever like them or get together with them."), or agreeing to choose an alternative neither would have chosen on his or her own ("You want a vacation on the beach and I want a vacation in New York City, so we'll go somewhere neither of us would have imagined—biking from inn to inn in the Pacific Northwest.").

---

**TIP:** Relationships in which disagreements or arguments are resolved with mutual satisfaction—not giving in or settling—have greater contentment and longevity.

---

Observation of couples shows three basic approaches to handling conflict. These are exemplified by couples who

- argue heatedly, then "kiss and make up";

- talk everything through calmly, never seeming to disagree or argue;

- have two different styles of fighting or disagreeing and often end up hurt, angry, and with issues left unresolved until they learn a mutual way to resolve their disagreements.

If you and your partner have a similar style of handling conflict, then you will probably be more effective in resolving disagreements. If, on the other hand, you have a dissimilar way of approaching conflict, then you may experience difficulty reaching a resolution.

Let's look at an example of each of these three approaches to conflict listed on the previous page.

## The Connected Fighters Who "Kiss and Make Up"

Wally and Bette are an example of couples that argue heatedly, then kiss and make up. Wally and Bette have been married for more than twenty-six years. They met in high school, married in their early twenties, and have successfully raised four children, who are now ages eighteen to twenty-five. While their house may be a bit on the messy side—with dogs, cats, and art and work projects in every room—there is a palpable warmth, generosity of heart, and playfulness that is contagious when you are around this ebullient couple and their highly interactive family. When asked how they have managed to build such a solid relationship, Bette and Wally share what they feel is a key ingredient. Bette said "We were drawn to each other right from the start," and Wally added, "I loved her energy, lack of self-consciousness, and ability to have a good time even when doing serious things. We're both like that."

However, things don't always run smoothly. Bette continued, laughing heartily,

> That part of our relationship has been one-half of the equation. And the other half is that we fight! That's right, we fight. Good old out-and-out loud voices, lots of opinions, both having our total say—maybe nobody listening.

Wally agreed,

> It's all but the kitchen sink. The kids know enough to get out of Mom and Dad's way and mind their own business. It's all but throwing pots and pans around here for a few minutes. But then it's over. Things get real quiet for a half hour or so, and then she gets real sweet to me.

Bette chuckled, taking the bait playfully.

> You're right. I like a good row, but then I love to kiss and make up. He doesn't do so bad himself!

Bette and Wally exemplify the couple that fights, comes to resolution, and then kisses and makes up. If both you and your partner handle conflict this way, it might work for you most of the time. It will work if you maintain the 5-to-1 positive-to-negative ratio and you fight fairly or respectfully. Wally and Bette learned to do this using the 10 Steps. As Wally explained,

> When the kids were little, we fought and made up the same way, only we were more hurtful in what we said. We didn't even remember the words, but one of our eldest kids Mickie did, and he asked if we were going to get a divorce or something bad. We realized we had to be careful or the kids would get the wrong impression.

Bette clarified,

> We didn't want them to be afraid, because we knew there was no way we were going to split up. We're just noisy people! What worked, and what we've continued to use, are the Big Picture Partnering skills. I think we had three coaching sessions and it's worked ever since.

Wally and Bette then explained which Big Picture Partnering skills they use to this day—and every day—to balance their loud and boisterous style of conflict. Said Wally,

> I think about the rules for fighting almost every day. First, we stopped saying hurtful things and stopped swearing at each other when we were yelling. Then, we naturally kiss and make up and get back to our usual interaction—which is darn fun most of the time. If ever one of us is down, we may just give a bit more than normal and usually we bounce right back. We naturally do lots of nice things for each another and that is the key. We are stuck to each other. What we've got going is like glue. Nobody's going anywhere.

Bette went on,

> We explained that to Mickie and the other kids. Now they just roll their eyes and know we'll get over it whenever we start to argue. They trust that we are a family. They see us fight, but they also see lots of kisses, hugs, banter, and loving between us. They know we are solid, and so are they.

Wally added a final note:

Yeah, the kids also have developed this style of arguing then making up—not surprising with us as parents! All of them have agreed, at one time or another, that they'd rather grow up in a lively household like ours than in a quiet home where you can't tell if people really love each other.

## The Rational Discussants

Let's look at another couple with a totally opposite style of dealing with conflict: You may recognize yourself as you listen to Ned and Arlyce who never yell or holler. They represent the couple that both talk calmly during a disagreement. Don't be fooled. This does not mean that calm, quiet types don't have issues—sometimes they just go quietly under the rug! Ned and Arlyce scored themselves as 50 percent Traditional-Merged, and 50 percent Big Picture Partnering when they first came in for counseling. I had to ask if they ever fought or disagreed. Arlyce acknowledged,

> Actually, we disagree quite a lot. We have differing political views, thoughts about how people should act, and even some interesting philosophical differences about the meaning of life.

Ned agreed,

> We just aren't the kind of people who get very loud or angry when we disagree. I think our families influenced us both. Both sets of parents really respect one another's points of view and have serious debates about religion, philosophy, and politics, even the weather! It was the way we had family discussions at the dinner table almost every night.

Arlyce informed me,

> We even met in college debate class. We simply discuss things, talk until we both have been listened to, and then move on. I know some couples might find it tedious to talk as much as we do, but we both enjoy lots of verbal interaction. It is intellectually stimulating and it makes the two of us feel close.

Ned concluded, with a nod and a chuckle,

I know Arlyce really loves me because she listens to everything I have to say, and I have a lot to say! I try to do the same for her. Not many other women would be so interested in all my thoughts—magnificent or irrelevant!

On the other hand, behind this calmer style of conflict, in which voices are never raised and both partners listen to the others' words, there were issues they had simply avoided and that were left unresolved. They gradually admitted that even their style of discussion did not encourage them to always say what they thought, felt, or wanted about topics like their waning sex life or how they needed to shift their finances to prepare for retirement. They knew they needed to become better partners and face some of these issues together and quickly learned to apply their calm style of disagreeing to these issues. As they shared their thoughts and feelings about sex and money, it became apparent they could no longer act so Traditional, and they became less Merged. They continue to develop their Big Picture Partnership, visiting with me very infrequently when they find themselves avoiding any issue.

## The Mixed Contenders

Now let's turn to a relationship in which each partner has a different way of dealing with conflict. Darla and Isaiah have been together for six years. This is how Isaiah described their different styles:

I love her, but I'm getting worn down. Darla is always on my case. It seems like everything becomes a big issue, and she has to talk about it. After awhile, I just tune her out. I don't want to. It wasn't like this before we moved in together. I made her happy back then, I guess.

Darla sputtered, trying to explain her side of the story to me—almost in tears—with anger brimming under her words:

You used to listen to me, or so I thought. Now, you walk out of the room! You won't talk to me! I get so frustrated. If only he knew that if we just talked about it we could easily clear the air and I'd be happy. I know it seems like I'm always upset with him about something—but it's because he won't talk to me! If he talked we'd get over it quickly. I just know we would.

Isaiah retorted quietly,

> I can't help it. If you'd just calm down, maybe I could think. Did it ever occur to you that I'd come talk to you? But my mind goes blank. I end up feeling stupid and belittled by you. I saw my mom treat my dad that way. It took me a long time to realize she was just as frustrated as my dad was when he would roll his eyes and walk away from her. I guess maybe my mom and Darla are both hurting, but I can't stand the yelling and don't know how to get her to calm down.

Darla and Isaiah were both hurting. They had everyday issues they disagreed about and could not resolve because they could not talk about them in an effective way. On top of that, they felt alienated and angry at each other's way of dealing with conflict. The longer this went on, the more they both felt misunderstood and unloved. If you have differing styles of fighting or disagreeing, you probably aren't able to effectively resolve your conflicts. If this is the case for you and your partner, the two of you will need to learn a safe and mutually agreed upon style for resolving conflicts.

Darla and Isaiah are a common and classic example of a couple in which one person avoids conflict and the other person appears to seek engagement or conflict. When you mix these two styles of dealing with conflict, it can seem like trying to mix oil and water.

A regular complaint among couples like Darla and Isaiah is that one spouse is more verbose, explosive, or needs to talk a problem through "right now," while the other spouse leaves the room or grows as silent as a brick wall. If the more verbally aggressive partner goes on for too long, sometimes the quieter person explodes. Such a response can lead to more verbal assaults on the part of the aggressive partner; or it may result in the quieter partner having an uncharacteristic rageful outburst to get the needed "space" by causing the verbal partner to go away hurt and confused. Couples like this often end up in stalemate. Disagreements pile up—unresolved. If this kind of interaction goes on for too long, issues hang heavy around their relationship, like threatening dark clouds. As Dr. John Gottman's research would note, these couples are more likely to break up, especially because the positive interactions often do not outweigh the negative.

Darla and Isaiah were skeptical that any kind of intervention would help their relationship, but they were anxious to try something new. Isaiah said,

> I just don't want to throw away the last six years and then find out we could have fixed it. I know there must be things we both can learn to change.

Darla agreed,

> Even if we do break up or never get married, at least we'll know why. At least, that's what I'm hoping for.

In relationships like Darla and Isaiah's, issues go unresolved for months or even years, yet the couple continues to use the same old style of arguing. When they want to learn how to partner, the first requirement is that they agree to stop fighting—just like you have been instructed to do. This gives you time to nurture the good feelings (Step 1), practice regular talking (Step 2), and implement the other 10 Steps of Big Picture Partnering. You want to be on the same team—more connected—so you can tackle the issues together. Otherwise, you are simply tackling and hurting each other with your blame and disappointment. When couples fight over and over about the same issues, continuing to fight is surely not going to work! The Do Not Fight Pact is for the short term so couples can shore up positive feelings and experiences. Typically, couples who fight a lot are so worn out and so relieved not to fight anymore that they willingly agree—with the caveat that they will talk about the disagreements, but only when they both feel safe and are able to communicate respectfully.

Darla and Isaiah had been fighting for some time. They agreed to stop fighting while they assessed their relationship style and began to increase the positives between them. Then they spent the next few months implementing all 10 Steps and learning how to handle conflict in a way that was new for both of them, in a way that was safe, effective, and mutually beneficial. They practiced taking *time-outs*—which you will learn about later in this chapter—when a discussion became too heated. They agreed to come back to discuss issues in a mutually calm and respectful way later. Darla learned that, given time and space and with a gentler and less angry approach on her part, Isaiah would tell her what was on his mind. She had to slow down. Isaiah had to learn to speed up his response time a bit and risk talking to Darla.

In the beginning, Darla and Isaiah scheduled regular talking time for twenty to thirty minutes every other day. They practiced actively listening to each other. Gradually they used all 10 Steps. As they practiced, they got rid of misunderstandings and assumptions. They each felt more listened to and more loved. Major areas of conflict became mutually workable and they became more creative problem solvers. They still did not agree on everything, but then, no two people do. Instead, they engaged in understanding each other's point of view. How did they feel about making this change? Darla said,

It never occurred to me how much I was assuming about Isaiah's point of view—on everything! I used to listen to him and felt we were pretty similar. Now when I stop to actually listen to him again, I don't always find that we agree on something, but I do feel connected. I've listened with an open heart and without judgment, so I now understand his point of view. And he's listening more to me. I feel understood. It's funny how being listened to is much more important now than having him always agree with me.

Isaiah gave Darla's hand a squeeze. He said jokingly,

I agree. We know that she's not always right! No, seriously, we are just much more respectful. I have learned not to run away from her anger. She still gets upset with me, but I can hear her now. When something bothers one of us, we ask to talk. If we can't do it then, we make a time later. At first it took a much longer time to talk things through. Now that we've cleared the air on the big things, a disagreement may take five or ten minutes to talk through.

Darla added,

This leaves us lots more time for the pleasurable things we both enjoy. It's more like when we first met. I think we both have tapped back into the reasons we were drawn together.

Once Darla and Isaiah sorted through the unresolved issues that they categorized as daily details, they went on to envision their Big Picture dreams. They put their creativity toward planning their wedding, purchasing a new home, and preparing themselves for the family they both wanted. They continue to use the 10 Steps and especially the Intentional Dialogue (see Step 9) when they are in conflict. As their problems subsided, they used all 10 Steps to work toward their dreams together. Darla exclaimed,

To think that we almost broke up six years ago, before we learned Big Picture Partnering! Two kids, happy jobs, and a calm home life are our reward.

Isaiah concluded,

I know we have the skills to continue to develop contentment in the coming phases of our life together—as the kids get older and as we get older. It's a good feeling to be successful—not perfect, by any means—but successful, and not only at work, but also with each other and our family.

Just like Darla and Isaiah, once your daily details are running smoothly, you will apply this same Big Picture approach to bigger goals and future dreams.

If you were fighting a lot prior to starting this approach, and if you are still in continuous conflict and have not been able to implement Steps 1–5, I encourage you to consider seeking a good therapist, marital counselor, coach, peer mentor, or educator. Such expert guidance will help the two of you sort through your difficulties. Then you will be ready to use all 10 Steps and create the Big Picture you desire.

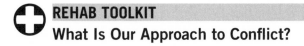

## REHAB TOOLKIT
## What Is Our Approach to Conflict?

Take a moment to reflect. Ask yourself the following questions: "What is my approach to conflict, disagreements, differences, or arguments? What is my partner's approach?" One or both of you may be loud, verbose, wanting to talk things through immediately. One or both of you may be calm, quiet, or even avoidant of conflict. How have your individual approaches to conflict worked or been harmful before you agreed to stop fighting in Step 1? Write the answers in your notebook.

Again, stop and reflect on how you and your partner handled conflict before beginning this program. How has your approach helped or hindered your sense of trust, openness, or safety between you? Is it the same for each of you, or is one of you feeling unsafe or untrusting? What do you think has caused this? How might you have contributed to these feelings between you? (Save your notes, as you will revisit these exercises later in this chapter.)

When you engage in Big Picture Partnering, you learn to see conflict from a new vantage point. Conflict is transformed from a battle between enemies into an opportunity to learn about each other's unique view of a situation and creatively solve problems together.

## Emotional Overload: How Time-Outs Can Be Helpful

Let's refer back to Darla and Isaiah and the common scenario in which one person is more verbose, maybe more explosive, and more insistent on his or her need for communication while the other person tends to shut down, become a brick wall or tongue-tied, or even walk out of the room when the partner is talking.

## Fight or Flight

The fight-or-flight response is an instinctual response left over from prehistoric days when our survival was dependent on our ability to run from disaster or overcome the threat through fighting. Built into each of our bodies is a tendency to do one or the other in the face of anything we feel is a threat. Now our response may be more exaggerated than the circumstance warrants, on the other hand, because this is an instinctual response, most often we cannot stop its onset right away. The fact that you or your partner has an instinct to flee the scene or feels threatened and has an instinct to fight back is no one's fault. It is important you both learn to how to step back, let the feelings of threat subside, and then come together in a calmer way.

Research has found that many men go into a fight-or-flight response in the face of certain kinds of communication. Using bodily measures such as electrodes, researchers have shown that some men actually become emotionally "flooded"—that is, they are not able to think. They sweat. Their hearts beat faster. They freeze or they want to run. Sometimes they fight back by verbally exploding in order to push the threatening situation or person away. While the researchers did not study this response pattern in women, I have noted this same fight-or-flight reaction in some women whose mates are more verbally aggressive and insistent.

Melody, for example, reported the following,

> I don't want to shut down, but Arnie's such a big guy, he has such big energy, and when he is upset about something he just talks and talks—at me. I get confused. I feel like he's right about some things, but I just can't think. I can't even respond, and that makes him even more upset. I end up physically drained and sometimes very depressed.

In the case of the previous couple, Darla and Isaiah, and the current couple, Melody and Arnie, the verbal partner needs to know the other partner does not shut down by choice. Rather, it is the body's instinctual response—a remnant from the times when we needed to physically flee from or fight back against threats to our very existence! That you or your partner has an instinct to flee the scene or feels threatened and has an instinct to fight back is no one's fault. On the other hand, if you are the more verbose, excitable, verbally insistent, or aggressive partner, you will not get what you want—you will not get your needs met—if you continue to use this approach with this particular type of mate.

If you are the one who flees or fights back when you feel pushed into a corner, you, too, are not getting your needs met. Your style is also ineffective. We all blow it once in awhile. We all get emotionally overloaded from time to time. Rather than judging your partner or yourself, it is important to keep focusing on how you can help yourselves to become more effective communicators and partners. When you are emotionally overloaded or heated, if you sense your Child Self or Critical Parent Self emerge, take a time-out. It is important to calm down and clear your mind. Then you can start afresh and communicate in a way that makes you feel effective and proud of both yourself and your partner.

## How to Take a Time-Out

Taking a time-out should to be OK in any relationship, but especially if you are building a rock-solid and successful Big Picture Partnership. Sometimes you require space. At times, you want to think. Occasionally, there is something else you need to attend to before you can work on resolving a problem with your partner. Sometimes you are shutting down and can't hear clearly or respond with grace and dignity. At others, one of you is talking too loudly, too emotionally, and ought to put the brake on—to step back and take a big, deep breath.

To have effective communication in stressful times, the time-out rules are as follow:

- If you feel you are verbally out of control or are shutting down and retreating, you are responsible for saying, "I need a time-out."

- Both partners must automatically agree to the other's need for a time-out—no questions asked, no further statements—even if doing so is frustrating.

- The person taking the time-out must come back to the discussion when he or she has agreed to and when both partners are calmer.

Initially, it may be difficult for either person to follow the rules of the time-out. If you know, however, that you have the option to make your communication more effective by taking or giving a time-out, it will make sense. Especially when two people agree to honor these time-out rules, they learn to trust that their partner

- won't give chase and demand to talk immediately;

- will come back and resume the conversation or resolve the issue when he or she feels calmer. The person taking the time-out must eventually resume the discussion and, if possible, say when a good time to talk will be. For example, "Honey, I am shutting down and need a time-out now, but I really want to talk about this. I need to go walk around the block. Let's talk about this . . . in an hour . . . this afternoon . . . tonight after the kids are in bed . . . tomorrow evening when I'm more rested."

In Big Picture Partnering, couples agree to come back to talk within one day.

Taking a time-out also allows partners to drop petty disagreements that arise. Sometimes, by the time they have resumed the discussion, neither can remember what they were fighting about. Occasionally, they have thought it through and can easily resolve the issue if it is small. When issues are complex or heated, I recommend holding off until both partners are calm. At that point they are ready to use the Intentional Dialogue technique you will learn in Step 9.

Let's summarize here. Healthy resolution is acquired when partners

- stop the arguments and fights that have not been working;

- follow basic respectful communication guidelines outlined at the beginning of this chapter;

- use time-outs as an effective means of stopping behavior that inhibits communication, such as shutting down or talking too heatedly;

- become trustworthy and accountable for resuming a discussion no matter which one initiated the time-out;

- agree to learn a mutual approach to conflict resolution (just as you will in the steps to come).

# ✚ REHAB TOOLKIT
## Step 6 Exercises

### *How Do You Currently Resolve Conflicts—and What Part Do You Play?*

In this chapter you began to reflect on how you and your partner resolve (or fail to resolve) conflicts. Continue to write in your notebook. Ask yourself, "How do we disagree?" Are bad feelings and needs left hanging in the air, clouding the good times between you? What is your approach to dealing with conflict? What is your partner's approach? (For example, do one or both of you yell, scream, holler, or "pursue" your partner for answers? Do either of you withdraw or feel defeated or overwhelmed?) Incorporate your earlier reflections on how these actions and feelings contribute to either of you feeling trusting, safe, and open.

Once you have identified your approaches to handling conflict, write about what you would like to change. Using the list of Common Communication Wisdom and Gottman's list of behaviors that promote marital success on pages 108–110, reflect on what you would like to do differently.

Before you discuss specific communication changes with your partner, take some time to reflect on your willingness to change your pattern of conflict and resolution. This is a hard one to face. We often want to blame the other person. Alternatively, we want to wait for the other person to change first. For example, we tell ourselves, "If only they'd stop yelling at me, then I'd come forth and give them a hug." Or, "If only they'd say something kind before telling me what they think I should do differently, it would be so much easier." What I'd like you to do here is consider *what you would have to do differently* to change the pattern of conflict resolution in your partnership. When you are ready, make a commitment to changing the part you play in arguments with your partner. Answer these four questions in your notebook to clarify this commitment:

1. "Am I committed to doing my part to communicate respectfully and effectively in disagreements with my partner? Am I willing to hold my tongue, if necessary? Am I willing to take time-outs if I need them? Am I willing to stay in my Adult Self in order to enhance our interactions?"

2. "What are four concrete steps I can take toward better resolving our disagreements, large or small?"

3. "How might I sabotage or get in the way of resolving disagreements effectively?"

4. "What am I willing to change, starting this week?"

## Your Desire to Resolve Conflicts

Now, spend time discussing these patterns of conflict and conflict resolution with your partner. You might wish to do this during regular talking time. Ask yourselves, "How do we resolve conflict now? What patterns emerge? How would we like to do things differently? Are we committed to continuing to learn all 10 Steps of Big Picture Partnering and using them to learn new ways of resolving our conflicts?" Share the changes each of you is willing to make. Take turns asking the four questions listed previously and listen to your partner's desire to change.

## Your Need for Time-Outs

Individually, reflect on the need for time-outs in your partnership. Does one of you storm out while the other wants to pursue the disagreement? On the other hand, are you both able to stay and discuss your differences respectfully? If not, would you be willing to take a time-out as a way to improve your communication?

Discuss this during your regular talking time. Make an agreement to follow the time-out rules (found on page 121) even if you only need them once in awhile. They are useful rules to have in your back pocket, especially during times of stress.

## Identifying Unresolved Issues

Spend some time on your own this week, writing in your notebook about areas in your partnership that you feel require change, creative problem solving, or improvement. What improvements would make your partnership stronger? Consider the details you deal with on a day-to-day basis, such as chores, finances, sexuality, schedules, kids' activities, adults' social activities, and so on, as well as larger issues such as the goals you aspire to, the dreams you shared when you first came together, and the desires you have for the years ahead. These goals and dreams may be lost in your day-to-day demands or disagreements. Do not share your thoughts right now; save your list or notebook notes for further exercises in Steps 7 and 8.

Chapter 9

# STEP 7:

## Put Your Issues on the Table so They Don't Come Between You

When couples have troubles, they typically do a lot of blaming and finger pointing. Each partner has the unconscious expectation that if their partner changed, everything would be fine in their relationship.

While there may be some element of truth when one person wants their partner to change, typically they are

- blaming their partner and creating a fight or pushing him or her away;

- not taking responsibility for their part in the problematic communication;

- not viewing the issues as a joint venture to be dealt with together.

In this chapter, while exploring **Big Picture Step 7: Put Your Issues on the Table so They Don't Come Between You**, you will

- learn the concept of "standing still" to stop old behaviors that aren't working;

- practice replacing your old behaviors with new ones by coming together versus taking sides;

- place your issues on your "partnering table" so they do not come between you;

- reflect on your willingness to come up with solutions that satisfy both of you—the win/win perspective.

This step will show you how to keep disagreements from coming between you or tearing you apart.

Earlier you signed the Do Not Fight Pact and agreed to discontinue fighting in the old way while you read this book. You adopted a partnering perspective, renewed your connection, and learned to talk and listen again. In the exercises for Step 1, when you signed the Do Not Fight Pact, you wrote down everything that seemed like an issue or unresolved problem at the time, and you tucked that list away to be used later.

All couples have disagreements and differences. All relationships experience problems. You cannot keep your problems or issues tucked away on a list. That was just for a time. Now it is time to learn and practice the proven ways that help partners to not only resolve conflicts together, but also to reach for their dreams together. Steps 7–10 will give you the mindset and the tools to clear up the problems on your lists and to work toward your goals together.

## Stand Still and Be Open to Change

In order to create change or a new way of relating to each other, in order to resolve the previously unresolved issues on your relationship table, you must stop using your old pattern. It's not working! Patterns are like habits. Some habits can be good, such as brushing your teeth or making your bed regularly. Some habits are simply not helpful, such as fights between you or seeing your partner as your enemy.

The good news is that both positive and negative habits are formed rather quickly. A habit is just a rut or a mental groove you are stuck in. For example, it's now common knowledge that it takes a mere twenty-one to thirty days to develop a new eating or exercise habit. You've already proven through your work in previous chapters how it only takes a little while to increase your positive-to-negative ratio and to talk and listen regularly. The same is true for repetitive negative interactions between you. If you are in a negative rut of bickering, fighting, or cold war silence, know that you can change this pattern in a short time. I'm going to show you how in the next few chapters. First, you must stop what you are doing that is causing you to be stuck. You do this by what I call standing still and, eventually, by trying something new.

*Do not fight* meant biting your tongue or walking away to focus on controlling your own negative responses. You probably needed that back in Step 1 as you started this program. *Standing still* is more advanced. It is an opportunity to reflect on your deeper intention (Do I really want to lash out and be cutting and sarcastic? Do I really think this man I've been married to for nine years is a jerk? Do I really want to hurt her feelings?) and pave ways for change, for new interactions (Maybe I could say "That made me feel like you don't care," rather than lashing out. Maybe I can remind him about the family birthday this weekend rather than assuming he's a selfish jerk. Maybe I can slow down and listen again because I know my ignoring her hurts her.) Your old ways keep you apart. Standing still opens the way for understanding and to come closer again.

Finances are one example of an important and often difficult issue for many partners to resolve. Richard and Katherine had many discussions, over the course of many months, regarding how to manage both individual and family finances. They've been together for two years and are engaged, with the wedding one year off. Paying for their wedding is a mutual goal for both Richard and Katherine but coming up with win/win ways of accomplishing this was a problem. Both Richard and Katherine had their individual ways of managing money, with Katherine being the one who held the purse strings closed, checking account balances daily and enjoying keeping five or six different savings accounts for everything from the wedding to vacation plans to holiday-gift savings. She was frustrated with Richard's more easy-going approach.

As Richard and Katherine worked toward becoming Big Picture Partners for life, they frequently squabbled; she blamed and criticized Richard, and he became sarcastic about her tight-fisted approach. For a number of months, they bickered constantly, not only about the wedding savings, but also about everything. Finally, they decided they needed to put their issues on the table and develop win/win solutions together.

Richard said,

> I realized I had been holding onto the notion that I was right and it was getting us nowhere. Even though I don't feel the need for as many savings accounts as Katherine, she is making fantastic progress in building our wedding savings, and I really do want to work on this together.

Katherine added,

While we haven't fully come up with a total financial approach that will work for all of our money in our marriage, when I stopped demanding that Richard do it my way and stopped feeling like he was the bad guy and chasing after him to contribute, he had time to come toward a calmer me. I stood still and just waited. It took about a week, and then he brought up the topic. He actually asked me how much I had put into the account and what his half would be. Whew! Was I ever relieved.

Richard then went on to explain how they established saving for the wedding as a mutual goal:

Then we really talked about how much we wanted the same things and needed to stop criticizing each other. We agreed that we don't know how to handle our finances when we are married, but we both want to contribute to this savings account now. We set up an automatic withdrawal from my account, and Katherine will simply track to see we are both contributing about equal amounts going forward.

Katherine said,

This wasn't easy, but we have both learned how our assumptions about each other's style of intentions were destructive. Keeping our issues on the table can save us a lot of heartache.

Richard added, "And it saved the time we spent bickering!"

What is important is that Richard and Katherine have learned to put issues on the table, stand still, and be in a win/win mindset as they approach anything together. It may take time, patience, and care to arrive at the mutual "yes!" but the feeling of well-being is definitely worth waiting for.

Just like in the example of Richard and Katherine, you can observe a pattern of how any two people come together or move apart over their differences. Each couple develops an intimacy distance they maintain throughout their relationship, unless they become aware of their old pattern and work to change it. Eileen McCann, in her book *The Two-Step: The Dance Toward Intimacy* (published in 1987 and still in print today) animated this intimacy distance and dance quite pointedly and often humorously in this thirty-minute read.

Ideally, partners should come together and move apart, come together and move apart with a nice rhythm; meeting in the middle and then taking private or individual time, then meeting in the middle again. The rhythm of the coming together and the moving apart can vary for each couple based on the intensity of the intimacy. For example, suppose a couple has deep, deep personal discussions that are very self-revealing early on as they fall in love. They may seek a little space to absorb the feelings these revelations engendered—not to disconnect but to be with one's self. Another example would be a deeply intimate sexual experience between two people who are tender and vulnerable, maybe even passionate or tempestuous. Their bodies and beings may need some time to absorb and enjoy both the pleasure and the powerful closeness. The same is true when a couple explodes in rage and says destructive things. The partners often retreat to their corners and may take days to reemerge and reconnect.

When couples are not doing well, you often see one of two patterns: either both people avoiding each other or one chasing and the other withdrawing. Sometimes, if the chase continues and feels like nagging or haranguing, the partner who is running away or withdrawing will decide he or she has had enough and will turn and snarl or fight back, causing the chaser to then shut down or flee. If you could see the intimacy-distance set up between the two, you would notice that they rarely get any closer or further away. One person is always being chased and the other is always chasing; one is always being pursued and the other is pursuing. In this relationship dance, these couples never get any closer until they learn new steps.

No matter which dance you and your partner have been executing and no matter how much intimacy-distance you have created between you, you can begin to change your pattern by standing still. That's right. It is similar to the notion of "fighting for now." Stop chasing. Stop pursuing. Stand still. You will have to face your own feelings and notice your own fears or frustrations.

For example, many women say,

> But if I don't talk to him, or beg him, or tell him what to do he might never talk to me.

Men often say,

> If I just stopped to listen to her, she might never be quiet. I might never please her.

Do you hear the fear of loss? Yet choosing, avoiding, or lashing out do not get you what you really want. So, stand still. Stop any old behaviors. What you do next

## ✚ REHAB TOOLKIT
## What Is Our Relationship Dance?

Stop for a moment and reflect on your pattern: When there are ill feelings, unresolved issues, or problems between you, which "dance" do you and your partner perform?

- Does one of you want to talk it over, while the other withdraws or goes silent? Do both of you end up feeling frustrated?

- Does one of you become defensive when an issue arises? Does that person lash out at the other to get him or her to stop talking about it? Do both of you end up frustrated?

- Do you both come out arguing and disagreeing, while no one is listening? Do you then end up frustrated?

- Do you both go silent and withdraw and then feel down or defeated?

- Do you push the topic under the rug and simply go on as though the bump under the rug is not there?

On your own, write about the pattern you see the two of you engage in when there are problems. You will return to these reflections in the exercises at the end of this chapter.

---

will depend on your situation, but standing still is a good start. It is a change. If your dance is not toward intimacy, you need change.

Chasing your partner will not reassure you. It does not teach you to trust that your partner will come toward you on his or her own—because of want, because of love.

For those of you who have been running away, withdrawing or avoiding, you will never find out if your partner calms down when you simply stand still and listen without trying to fix anything. He or she may not calm down entirely or be satisfied at first. You will have to learn to communicate more and resolve problems together, but standing still is a start.

As you become better at standing still, coming together versus taking sides in a conversation is a particularly useful tool.

## Come Together Versus Taking Sides

If you always take opposite points of view or if you are competitive or always polarize, practice replacing this behavior with actions that promote "coming together."

# ✚ REHAB TOOLKIT
## Practice Standing Still

As you reflect on your pattern, imagine standing still. When you and your partner are on the verge of an old negative behavior or a bickering and blaming session, you might practice biting your tongue. Then actually listen and say, "I hear you," instead of fighting back or disagreeing. You might invite your partner to take a walk. You might wash the dishes, scrub a floor, or clean a bathroom. Then you might come back to watch TV together without withholding attention or affection or holding a grudge.

The point is to *just to do anything except your old negative behavior* without judging you or your partner. Standing still and doing nothing is doing just that. Observe yourself while you stand still. Practice some deep breathing or count from one to ten if it buys you time or if standing still makes you feel afraid. Remind yourself that nothing worse can happen if you simply stand still, close your mouth, refrain from saying the same old things, or show a willingness to listen. As you practice standing still, you will gradually imagine a new positive behavior you could do instead. After a few mental rehearsals, you might try the new behavior you imagine.

If standing still does not work well the first few times, don't give up. Stay Adult. Eventually your partner will have to respond differently also. Most importantly, you may feel better about yourself. You are creating an opportunity for change, for new interaction.

---

I once assigned a particularly feisty couple the task of carrying squirt guns to remind them to "lay down their arms." They quickly learned to see the humor in how they approached each other as enemies rather than as allies. They had spent enormous amounts of time arguing over who was right and who was to blame. It had not only sucked up all their time and creative energy, but also it had polarized them so they could only see their differences. They guarded their individual turf very well, but they were unable to come together to resolve, build, create, or imagine anything new.

Relationships are not meant to be courtroom battles, war zones, or debate tournaments. Home should be a safe harbor where you can let your hair down, play, and be a little goofy. This behavior rejuvenates you for going back out into the world of work and high expectations—where sometimes battles do have to be fought. When we are competitive in the rest of our lives, learning to soften up when we walk in the front door takes practice. Of course you have differences. That is a given when two unique individuals spend time together. However, rather than oppose each other, why not actively seek common ground? When you focus on things in which you are similar, rather than in which you differ, you will

- both feel more accepted, listened to, and loved;

- establish an arena—rather than a boxing ring—in which to create what you both want in life.

## ✚ REHAB TOOLKIT
## Try Something New

Instead of your old negative response, you might say,

- "I hear what you are saying . . ."

- "Tell me more. That sounds interesting."

- "You sound excited (or sad or mad) about that. I'd like to understand what you are feeling."

If a verbal response feels awkward, you might do something physical: Sit near your partner on the couch, offer to bring a cup of coffee, ask if there's a chore your partner would like help with, or offer a hug or pat on the shoulder. Each of these can be a positive gesture, an olive branch, a coming together.

---

Think of yourselves as rivers flowing toward the equator, pulled by gravitational forces. Your individual waters flow in the same direction and seek a coming together—to form a larger, more forcefully flowing river or body of water. Your positive ideas, thoughts, dreams, conversations, and desires are like those waters seeking to merge—seeking to form a greater creative energy than either of you can manifest on your own.

Luis and Rosa had difficulty coming together. Rosa explained it this way:

We've been together for almost sixteen years. In the past, whenever I came up with an idea, Luis would either tell me about three or four better ideas he'd heard of, or describe all the problems we'd run into if we pursued my idea. As a result, we never went on any trips or took any classes together. It was hard to agree on how to socialize or do anything new. I always felt like he wanted to put a boulder in our path, like he didn't love me or want to support my ideas. I sort of felt like he thought my ideas were stupid.

Luis agreed they were having communication issues. He went on to explain the changes they were making:

Rosa is right. But I also thought she didn't support my ideas either. I would try to add my thoughts to hers when she came up with an idea, thinking it would help, but it never did. Instead, Rosa always felt like I was shooting her ideas down, or trying to promote my own ideas. When we were introduced to Big Picture Partnering, I learned to listen to Rosa first before injecting my suggestions. Once Rosa knew I had heard her, then she was open to hearing my additions. Gradually I realized that my whole family talks the way I used to! You say a thought or idea, and they take it in a million different directions, but never in the direction you had wanted. They forget to acknowledge your idea so you know you have been heard. Like me, they assume you know they have heard you by simply going on and injecting their thoughts. They don't even realize they are doing it—but nobody's ideas ever come together as a result.

As they learned to come together in their conversations, Luis and Rosa found that they resolved everyday problems more quickly and had fun more often.

## All Issues Go "On The Table"—Not Between You

Practicing standing still and adding new positive responses to your repertoire helps, but it does not take away those issues that remain unresolved. You may blame your partner for disagreements, differences, or even stressors from outside circumstances. When you blame your partner, you create a wall between you that cuts off your connection and feelings of closeness. You are no longer on the same team. You cannot work together to arrive at solutions. Putting your disagreements between you polarizes you. It is like being adversaries or enemies—at opposite ends of a tug-of-war rope. It may feel like a brick wall between you. It means you must adopt a new perspective. Put the issues on the table, so they do not blur or blind your vision or make you forget you are on the same team. Life is stressful enough without blocking out your partner and the lifeline of potential creative problem solving between you.

## Topics that commonly go on a couple's table include:

- Kids
- Work
- In-laws
- Household chores
- Holiday plans
- Couple dates
- Sex
- Religion
- Money
- Time commitments
- Schedules
- Problematic friends
- Social activities
- Retirement plans and dreams
- And so on

Examples of things that should go on your table include misunderstandings or disagreements between you or desires about any aspect of you life. These may include such things as differences in how each of you parent, desires for your family's happiness, or weekly squabbles over who should do the cooking or cleaning. Outside stressors that have an impact on you should also go on your table. These may include the emotional and financial ramifications of a difficult boss causing anxiety over job security. It may include a friend's breast or prostate cancer diagnosis causing you both to worry or grieve.

Anything that is a current or future need, a difference or disagreement, a desire or dream should go on your partnering table. Then the focus becomes, "How shall we handle this together?"

In Big Picture Partnering, all issues, desires, requests, differences, and disagreements go on the table rather than between you. All issues are viewed as simply life circumstances you address together. Then you work toward mutually satisfying solutions together. Refer back to the Figure on page 19 to visualize how this table is a forum for discussion of issues as you work toward new options and win/win solutions together.

## Make Win/Win Decisions Together

I've asked you to stand still and to practice some new behaviors that will be more constructive. You've been introduced to the idea of putting your issues and desires on your partnering table rather than between you. As you use your partnering table later in this chapter, you will reflect on your readiness to give up your own way and instead create win/win solutions together. This is the final aspect of Step 7: embracing the win/win mindset that is necessary for coming to mutually satisfying solutions to your differences or disagreements. You will practice this win/win mindset as you progress through all 10 Steps; this is a preview of the mindset Big Picture Partners remember and practice all of the time.

---

**TIP:** Big Picture Partnering is built on the notion that two people in a partnership should both come out winners. It recognizes the creativity within each partner and empowers both to work together to create win/win options that will work.

---

Working together for win/wins is the mark of a true partnership. Win/wins cannot happen when you put issues between you and blame, criticize, or demand. Win/wins also do not exist when there is too much compromising. When individuals over-compromise or shortchange themselves by abandoning their desires, they become resentful. Their identities and sense of self-worth are damaged.

In Big Picture Partnering there is no need to settle for less, because nothing goes into the Our World circle until you both fully agree to it. Some discussions are quick and easy; others may take days, weeks, or months to arrive at win/win decisions. If you are not reaching an agreement, then you may set the discussion aside for a while. Later you may revisit the topic, building on previous discussions until you have creatively and mutually arrived at a decision together.

In most relationships, minor differences of opinion or needs are easy to negotiate, with agreements going into the Our World circle. For example, take Mary and Tom's dinnertime discussion:

Mary: "Gee, honey, where shall we eat tonight? I think I'd like fish." Tom: "Actually, I feel more like steak." Mary: "Oh, you want steak? Well, what would you think about the surf-and-turf over at Clearwater Cafe?" If Tom doesn't want to go to the Clearwater Cafe, he might agree to have fish at another fish restaurant, because what he has to eat isn't really that important—he's just hungry. And, he's willing to wait until tomorrow night to grill steaks at home. He may also choose the good feeling he gets by pleasing his wife.

When it comes to topics with larger consequences, it is not good to compromise or settle too quickly. The following examples represent some topics that were complex and required time for each couple to arrive at solutions that would be satisfying to both partners. It required they keep the topic "on the table" and maintain a win/win mindset, while they listened for understanding and then creatively problem solved, as you will learn to do in the coming chapters.

Jo Ellen and Bradley struggled for months over Jo Ellen's dislike of Bradley's mother. This problem had an impact on holidays and time spent with her family versus his family. It also forced them to keep their in-laws on the table, so Jo Ellen was not disrespectful of Bradley still loving and caring about his mother, even though she did have irritating behaviors.

Blended families are always challenging. Tammy thought she knew this when she married Calvin, but his teenaged son's disrespect for household rules and their new relationship nearly broke them up. When they learned to put parenting on their partnering table and to come together around how to parent, this couple felt successful once again.

Another example is Heather, a savvy woman in her mid-thirties, recently married to Steve who is twelve years her senior. Heather really wanted a baby and was concerned that her age and health problems could affect conception. Steve also wanted a baby but was less tuned in to the biological clock. He thwarted deeper discussions, which made Heather angry. As they practiced partnering and put this and many other complicated issues on their partnering table, they were able to talk about the joys and difficulties they both anticipated in starting their family.

## ➕ REHAB TOOLKIT
## Step 7 Exercises

### *A New Way*

Earlier in this chapter you reflected on the pattern you fall into when problems arise. Now that you have completed the chapter readings, clarify your role in this pattern as you write in your notebook.

You have also imagined standing still and not following your old pattern. What have you imagined doing differently? Write about how you might interact with your partner in another way. Notice all the small ways you have made progress toward changing your part in sustaining the old pattern. Acknowledge your readiness to stand still, as well as any difficulties you may anticipate in doing your part differently, no matter what your partner does. Are there any new behaviors you have tried? If so, what has been the response? (Remember not to judge. Simply note the response and your need to stand still and try a new approach.)

In this chapter, you also reflected on your willingness to work together rather than have things go your way. In an earlier exercise, you put yourself in a mindset of new options neither of you may have thought of before. Reflect on your willingness to give up being "right."

Now, come together and discuss what you discovered about your

- willingness to put issues "on the table," not between you;

- ability to "stand still" rather that chase, avoid, pick fights, and so on;

- practice of replacing disagreements or silence with communication that promotes coming together and building on each other's ideas;

- desire to arrive at win/win solutions and your willingness to have things not go your way.

### Notice When You Polarize Versus When You Come Together

When you communicate with your partner, make a note of each time you find yourself pointing out differences, being negative about an idea, or taking an oppositional viewpoint. Write your observations in your notebook. Ask yourself, "What purpose do these polarizing comments serve for me? How can I break this habit? What do I need to do to better connect with my partner when we talk?"

## Practice Coming Together

As you raise your individual awareness of any polarizing behavior or negativity, consciously practice focusing your conversations on the ways in which you are similar or in agreement. Notice these especially during your regular talking times or in dialogue about your mutual goals.

Then, during one of your regular talking times, take turns describing what you have each noticed about the quality of your communication and how each of you is working to improve it. Be sure to show your appreciation for any progress you see the two of you making.

## What's on Our Table?

In this exercise you will revisit the lists you made and put away in Step 1 when you signed the Do Not Fight Pact on page 44 and in the Step 6 exercise Identifying Unresolved Issues on page 124. Before you share your lists and thoughts with your partner, first revisit your notes and reflect on which issues remain problematic or unresolved and which issues no longer seem to challenge you. Reflect on why some issues are no longer problematic to you. Write about what you are doing individually and together that has helped with these issues. Note when Steps 1–6 have either changed your behavior or your perspective on what seemed problematic.

Then come together and stay in a listening mode. Take turns sharing your lists and thoughts from these Step 1 and Step 6 exercises and your subsequent reflections on what has fallen away and what remains. Do not discuss or comment; simply listen to each other as you share the items that fall in two categories:

1. Those items that remain as issues or problems to be resolved, and anything that is a need for improvement, a desire, or a dream for you. (Remember to stay in the listening mode only. No discussion.)

2. Those items that no longer feel like issues to be overcome. (Listen to each other as you each share why these no longer feel like problems for you.)

Now refer to the diagram of your Big Picture Partnering table on page 19, and make two lists together. Make a list on your table of everything that is still an issue, desire, or dream for either or both of you. Then make a list of everything that has "fallen away" or everything that you have mutually resolved as you have worked through this book. Describe to your partner why you feel these previous issues are no longer concerns for you now. (Save these lists to be used in Steps 8–10.)

Then, review your list of issues that have fallen away and share which Big Picture tools you used to make them less problematic for each of you. Review the checklist of the seven steps you have learned so far (see box on the next page) and reflect together on the impact your partnering has made in helping you naturally resolve some of your issues.

Agree to work closely together as you learn a new way of resolving issues and finding creative solutions to your goals in the remaining chapters.

If none of your issues has been resolved at this point, do not worry. Simply share the list of things that are on your table to address as you continue to work through this program. Then review the checklist of Big Picture Steps and discuss how you are practicing each step individually and together. Are there any ways you can work more closely toward your goal of becoming Big Picture Partners?

## Checklist of Essentials Learned so Far:

**Step 1:** Increase the Positive Between You

**Step 2:** Talk Regularly and Take Turns Listening

**Step 3:** Deepen Your Individuality to Strengthen Your Relationship

**Step 4:** Discover the Depth of Your Commitment

**Step 5:** Address Any Issue Together—Whether It's Yours, Mine, or Ours

**Step 6:** Understand How You Manage Conflict

**Step 7:** Put Your Issues On the Table so They Don't Come Between You

Congratulate yourself and each other for the progress you have made from Step 1 until now, Step 7. Do something enjoyable together when you complete this chapter's exercises.

**Chapter 10**

# STEP 8:

## Turn Problems into Mutual Goals and Work Toward Them Together

Throughout this program you have discontinued fighting, changed your perspective, replaced negative interactions with positive ones, and become closer again. Along the way, you have identified unresolved issues, and you have reflected on things you'd like to improve or dreams you'd like to reach for. In Step 7, you made a master list and put it "on your partnering table." This list included every issue either of you felt was still unresolved, any areas needing improvement, and any other desires or dreams you long for.

Now, in **Big Picture Step 8: Turn Problems into Mutual Goals and Work Toward Them Together**, you are going to turn your problems into goals you can reach for together. You are going to turn what has been negative into a positive. The following is a list of what you will do:

- Turn your "issues and problems" into "daily details" you resolve together. Resolving everyday conflicts, or smoothing out your daily details, will be your primary focus in Steps 8–10. These are typically the everyday things that you bicker about or push under the rug and continuously trip over (such as child care or parenting differences, household chores, who plans the dates or social calendar, frequency of sex, how finances are handled, and so on). Because you encounter these differences, disagreements, or issues frequently, they can easily erode the good feelings between you. Addressing each one together will make your daily life run much more smoothly, freeing more time and energy for the next type of goal.

- Revitalize your Big Picture Dreams and reach for them together. These goals include bigger dreams and future desires. You may want to achieve some of these in three months and others in three, ten, or fifteen years. These Big Picture Dreams include goals that may feel a bit out of your reach and may take a bit longer to accomplish. So it is important to begin taking action toward achieving them gradually over time. Some of you are more ready to tackle your Big Picture Dreams than others. It doesn't matter. I want each of you to begin practicing envisioning your Big Picture Dreams and taking small steps toward achieving them together in the chapters ahead.

## Do You Have Experience with Goal Setting?

You may already be an active goal-setter. Perhaps you are one of those people who doesn't like or know how to set goals. The facts are

- people who set goals achieve more in life;

- when two people try to accomplish something together, they need to choose the same target and synchronize their efforts;

- those who clarify what they want and decide how they will work to achieve their dreams will do just that.

If you are not in the habit of setting goals, try the exercises in this chapter and experiment so you can measure the positive changes you create together as you go forward using the Big Picture approach. If you already have experience with goal setting, your focus will be learning to synchronize your goals and achieving them together as partners. Matching your goals and accomplishing them together will make you feel competent and successful as partners. You will become masters at achieving your own destiny—staying connected, having more fun, and being creative—far beyond the last page of this book.

## Your Goals: Are They Basic Needs, Desires, or Dreams?

As you grow, you each have the opportunity to provide for yourself and others at two levels. The first is a basic survival level. These are needs for food, clothing, shelter, and medical attention, as well as the money to attain these necessities. You also have sexual needs. The second level involves things you want. You do not need that red dress or new car, but you may want it! Unlike survival needs, which, if unmet, can result in illness or even death, wants can be modified. You may want a feast, but a steak sandwich may do. You may want a two-week vacation, but a day by the lake may better fit your schedule and budget—and give you the downtime you want.

Then there are the "wants" that some people think of as abundance or "havingness." Achieving a sense of simplicity and living a sustainable lifestyle falls into this category for some. For others, it is multiple homes, cars, and vacations. For yet others, abundance includes feeling at peace, being healthy, and having time for family and friends. Allowing yourself this kind of wealth may or may not involve money. Such abundance may relate to your wealth of knowledge, wisdom, friends, or laughter or your connection to God, a Higher Being, nature, or beauty. Allowing yourself to explore what you truly want is where your dreams and desires come into play.

Harry and Sue and Hans and Olivia are examples of couples who learned how to turn their problems and dreams into goals they accomplished together. Harry and Sue's daily details constantly tripped them up. By turning these hassles into goals, they were able to save their marriage. Once Hans and Olivia's daily details were smoothed out, they were ready to focus on a Big Picture Dream they'd had since early in their marriage.

Harry and Sue were desperate when they began to learn Big Picture Partnering. Married for five years with a sixteen-month-old baby, a three-year-old toddler, and a budget stretched thin in spite of two full-time jobs, they were constantly overwhelmed and stressed. They blamed each other and their bond was frayed. Sue said,

> If it weren't for the kids, we probably would have divorced a while back even though we love each other deeply.

Harry added,

That's for sure! We were totally unprepared for the demands of adulthood when we married in our early twenties and started having babies. Keeping house, buying groceries, cooking, cleaning, and paying the bills seemed like a cakewalk before Josie and Andy came along. I guess we both missed the role modeling of how to juggle all aspects of family life while going to work full time.

Eager to get out of their crisis, Harry and Sue worked hard to stop blaming each other. They turned their complaints into mutual goals they worked toward together—smoothing out their household organization, coming together on parenting styles, reworking home and office schedules, and creating a realistic budget they both honored. As Sue explained,

It was so hard at first to think of a problem as a positive goal we could work for, but once we figured out how to do it, it was almost a pleasure. We were no longer rageful or silent or hurting because we put our smarts toward saying what we wanted instead of saying what was wrong.

Harry piped in,

What a relief that lesson was! Instead of saying to Sue as I barged in the door after work, "Why the hell did you have to use the credit card again and don't you know that the checking account is also overdrawn?!" and Sue shooting back, "Well if you had to buy the groceries and feed this family, and if you'd only get that raise . . ." and our entire evening being destroyed, we practiced biting our tongues. Then we took the scary, painful step of sitting down— often at first, then less frequently as things got better—to listen to what each other "really" wanted.

Sue added,

Yeah. It was pretty basic. At first we learned to say "I need your help with the grocery shopping and the dishes." Or, "Could you pick up the kids from daycare one day a week so I could go workout before coming home to make dinner?" Or, "I'm worried about our debts and really want us to get our finances under control. Let's figure out a way to do this."

Harry built on Sue's thought,

Those basic needs turned into goals like, "We agree to develop a clear budget and stick to it." Then we identified what we needed to do to accomplish that goal. Our action items included downloading QuickBooks, hiring someone to help set it up, and inputting six months of data from our financial accounts. Then we had a clear picture of our spending habits.

Sue added with a laugh,

Yeah, both good and bad! Seeing it so clearly helped us talk about next action steps including where to cut back and where to save. It was hard, but I think we both felt very mature as we gradually got our finances under control and found new ways to have fun that don't cost as much. Being home in the evenings is also more pleasant so spending doesn't have to fill that void.

Harry finished their story by saying,

Now that we had completed that financial goal we have made new ones for this year: look into the kids' college fund, buy more life insurance and redo our will, and put more money toward retirement. We've done this same goal setting/goal accomplishing process with each and every one of our issues over the past three years. It saved our marriage and there is no way I'm stopping this partnering now!

Hans and Olivia are an example of a couple with some experience in goal setting in their work lives, who sought to apply these skills to becoming Big Picture Partners. Like Harry and Sue, they initially applied their goal setting to daily details, especially sharing household chores and coordinating many extended family activities. Married a second time, for six years, Olivia was a nurse who preferred to spend her free time spinning wool and making the weavings she took to craft fairs and sold at local gift stores. Hans would tell you he was "a techie nerd" who had worked for the same large corporation for many years. Nothing made him more content than having spare time to play computer games. Olivia would weave in the same room. But the housekeeping and the finances went neglected!

As they focused their new partnering skill on rectifying their most problematic areas, Hans and Olivia quickly became ready to dream their bigger goals. Already in their mid-forties, they decided to simplify their cleaning and financial routines until those were under control. Then they joined a Big Picture couple's workshop in which they shared their larger dream. They wanted to move to the country and purchase a small hobby farm where Olivia could raise the sheep for her wool and grow the herbs and flowers she enjoyed.

Olivia offered,

> We had looked at property earlier in our marriage, when this dream was alive and fresh. Over the years, nothing seemed within our price range or close enough to family, and our dream faded. But partnering opened up creativity we had forgotten about.

Hans and Olivia developed a solid Big Picture Partnership. They started by working on their daily details. Once their "house was in order," their creative juices flowed right into planning the life they had once dreamed of—before the dream was buried. This can happen for you, too. I have seen couples make monumental creative leaps in their lives, doing things they at first thought almost impossible. Olivia and Hans are one couple with a creative story to tell. Said Hans,

> I was totally unconvinced that we would ever move from the city, just because I work for a big technical company and couldn't imagine what I would do living on a farm. But as we talked and listened and explored and experimented with ideas and plans, and looked at property, and talked to other people, it all started to seem more possible—all except my work!

Olivia recalled,

> I remember all of our friends had to almost force you to talk to your boss about telecommuting. And he agreed almost immediately! You were so surprised!

Replied Hans,

> It's true. My boss said yes on the condition I'd come in to the office two days a week—and again, that seemed like an obstacle to me. But working as a team and exploring options kept us open to possibilities, and wouldn't you know, this farm came available three months later and we moved shortly after that.

Olivia said,

I love living in the country. We are close to Hans's parents, who are getting older, and he stays in the city one night a week and works from home the remaining time. It's as close to our ultimate dream as anyone can get!

Through their mutual efforts—learning to partner well, then applying their skills to daily details that bogged them down—Hans and Olivia unleashed their creative energy and resurfaced a dream from their early years. Hans and Olivia now share the life of their dreams, living in the country, creating art, and telecommuting. You can envision your goals and achieve your dreams as well.

## Turning Your Problems into Goals You Accomplish Together

In Step 1, you agreed to stop fighting and you put all your differences, disagreements, conflicts, and unresolved problems on a piece of paper and put it away. Then in Step 7, you put those same issues onto your partnering table rather than between you. You revisited your prior list and reflected on which issues still seemed to be problematic or unresolved. Then you came together and made a master list of everything on your table. You listened carefully to each other's concerns and desires as you combined your lists.

Now it is time to take out that master list of things you still need to change and turn former problems into mutual goals. In this step you will practice the mutual goal setting that will focus your efforts as you apply Steps 9 and 10. Each goal you state together will become a target toward which you aim your joint efforts. These joint efforts will help you find mutually satisfying, creative, win/win solutions—together.

You will also explore some Big Picture Dreams and put those back on your partnering table to envision and work toward. As you continue to partner and become masters of achieving your goals in the years to come, you will have fewer daily details that need to be smoothed out and more Big Picture Dreams on your goal list.

---

**TIP:** For every problem or obstacle, there are at least twenty solutions you can imagine. That is creativity.

---

There are many times in life when we have a desire and we talk ourselves out of it:

- "Oh, I'll never find the time."

- "I could never do that!"

- "Other people are able to do it, not me."

- "I don't have the money or the resources or the support or the _____."

- "We'll never resolve that issue or problem."

On it goes. Some people have an inner censor so powerful they don't even know they have dreams or desires. Some feel like a failure so they don't deserve to have a dream, even a little one.

Take a moment and read the paragraph below. Then close your eyes and visualize the scenario it describes.

> You are walking contentedly along a path. Off in the distance is a beautiful mountain peak surrounded by a sunny glow. Imagine that this peak is your greatest vision of what your life could become. Then as you walk step by step along your path, you suddenly come across a deep chasm, so deep it almost frightens you. Let's call this chasm "fear" or "obstacle" or "self-doubt" or "lack of deserving" or "too busy" or "too little money" or anything else that comes to your mind.

Know in your heart-of-hearts that here you are in danger of forgetting. You could forget that you have set your sight on the mountain peak, and this is simply a chasm. It is simply an obstacle. It needn't stop you. What you truly seek is ahead.

Now is the time to become creative in your visualization. Don't allow your fears and doubts to take center stage. Maybe you can build a bridge or fly an airplane across the divide or ride a donkey around it. Or perhaps some other idea may come to you.

Then breathe quietly as you reflect on how you sometimes forget that your dreams are at the top of the mountain peak and that the abyss is merely an obstacle to be gone around. Be like water and move around the problem, the obstacle, or the impediment. Don't let it stop you from moving step-by-step toward your dreams.

## Put Your Doubts Aside

Doubts are simply obstacles. For example, a potential obstacle to a short-term daily detail might be your disbelief that your husband would ever agree to cook twice a week or plan an entire date night for the two of you—including hiring the babysitter—so you dismiss your desire without writing it on your list. Your Big Picture Dream may be traveling to China at the end of next year, but you have no idea if your partner would like to go, how you will pay for it, or how to navigate this foreign country and language. However, if you put this goal on your list, it becomes a target toward which you will be pulled—you'll become aware of action items you can carry out to prepare yourself for such a trip. You will talk about your desire with your partner. Both of you may start to explore the local Chinese markets, buy maps and travel books about China, create a savings account for your trip, talk to travel agents or explore online, and so on. Before you know it, what once seemed an impossibility might be a reality!

In the following exercises you will turn your problems or issues, your dreams and desires into realistic, practical goals. You will start by setting goals you can accomplish within a three-to-twelve-month period. This is the beginning of a lifetime process if you are Big Picture Partners. In the final steps of this program, you will learn additional tools to turn your conflicts into creative solutions and help you reach for your dreams together.

Big Picture Partners schedule time to revisit their goals, give progress reports, or brainstorm and problem solve together. Whenever a goal is accomplished, couples celebrate and cross it off their list and then add a new one. Other couples revisit their goals together on an annual basis, for example, near the New Year or a wedding anniversary.

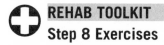

## REHAB TOOLKIT
## Step 8 Exercises

### Develop Your One-Year Goals

In Step 8 exercises, each of you will privately spend time writing your lists of Individual, Couple, and, if applicable, Family goals in your notebook. These goals are the things you wish for and want to accomplish in the coming year. As you work through the exercises, do not share your goals until instructed to. This first articulation of your goals is just for you. These lists may take you a few sittings to complete, so work on them a few hours at a time and then return to add additional thoughts after you have had time to reflect.

A good suggestion is to remember to write your goals in positive terms: Say what you want instead of what is wrong. For example, instead of saying, "I want us to stop fighting and arguing every night when we get home from work," you might say, "I'd like our evenings to be peaceful. I'd like some time to decompress and play with the kids when I get home. I'd like to reconnect with Sarah and I'd like to find out how she feels about meal preparation and putting the kids to bed, so we can work together to have a nice home life."

Another suggestion is to start with your global intention or desire and then become more specific. For example, you may state your global intention as a desire to be healthy. Then you would expand your intention into a goal: "My goal is to continue to be healthy by remaining active, eating more healthy foods, getting back into exercise, and losing some weight." Becoming more specific, you would flesh out action items and a timetable for accomplishing your goal by saying, "Starting in February, I will go back to the gym three times each week. I'll work out a schedule with Pam so I can come home an hour later on those days, and I'll offer to trade other times so she can also workout while I watch the kids. I'd like to lose ten pound in the next six months and I know Pam would, too. I'd like to work out a shopping/meal plan with her that will help us both to reach this goal if she's willing." For some intentions, you may not be able to write a specific goal at first. In addition, for some stated goals you may not know any action steps you might take today. Put them on your list of desires anyway. Over time you will add to your list on a regular basis—expanding your goals and accomplishing action items.

Your Individual Goals are what you'd like to accomplish personally this year: These goals may involve your work, your health, etc. Then, think about how you want your relationship to be one year from now. These are Couple Goals. Finally, what do you desire for your entire family? If you have children, these are your Family Goals. (This might include vacations and activities together, spending time learning something new as a family, and so on.)

To help you write these one-year goals, think about the goals you'd like to set in every area of your life:

- Your partnership

- Parenting

- Extended family

- Friendships

- Social life and activities

- Work life

- Spiritual life

- Creative pursuits

- Physical health, exercise

- Sex life

- Finances and investments—short term and long term

- Everyday household upkeep and maintenance

- Household projects, renovation, or remodeling

- Intellectual or learning activities

- Fun and leisure

- Travel

- Other

---

Give yourself some time, in a particularly nice setting, to consider these aspects of your life. Go somewhere overlooking a lake, curl up in your favorite chair, or take yourself out to your favorite coffee shop for a few hours. Take a written list of the above categories and any others that fit your circumstances.

Then start to write about what you need or want, fleshing out each of the categories on your list. Include

- things you already do and want to continue ("I like how we are parenting. I want to continue being a good father.");

- things you wish to resolve or change between you ("I want to improve our sex life and become more affectionate once again.");

- things you want to add or create ("We've never talked about our future dreams for twenty years from now. We need to start planning for retirement. I want to figure out a way to dream and make it financially feasible together." Or, "We need more couple time. I'd like us to have three short vacations this year, without the kids.").

Some people write a few paragraphs describing their overall goals or what they project their lives will feel and look like in one year. Others make lists.

Be sure to include all the little and big things that you desire to manifest in the coming year. You may wish to group these into short-term goals (one to three months) and longer-term goals (four to twelve months). For example,

- "I want a weekend vacation, alone with my husband, without the kids, next summer. We need some time on our own."

- "I want to start looking for a new job in six months, once I have learned what I set out to learn at this company. I need to talk to my partner about this."

- "I want us to continue practicing being more emotionally mature. I want us to continue becoming better communicators. I want us to feel more connected to each other by this time next year."

- "I want us to find a way to resolve disagreements about the children's bedtime and discipline. I'd rather spend our evenings relaxing and talking together."

- "I want to continue sticking to my budget and even have money saved by the end of the year. I would feel proud of myself if I accomplished that. It would contribute to our partnership."

- "I want to resolve our lack of sexual intimacy. We seem to be going through the motions these days."

- "This summer I want more time to golf or fish."

- "I want to feel closer to God. I'd like to talk more about our spiritual life."

- "I want to spend more time with my parents now that they are getting older and less active. I'm not sure how to balance this with my family, but I'd like my partner to support me in this."

Then circle or star your top three to four priority goals in the Individual, Couple, and Family goals categories. Here's an example of a fully thought-through individual intention, stated as a positive goal, fleshed out in action steps with a thorough timetable:

> During the coming year, my vision is to develop a better balance between personal, family, and work time. I am committed to experimenting with a few options toward accomplishing that goal. One is to go in to the office one hour earlier three days a week, close my door for that hour, and use that quiet time to get through my paperwork. This will enable me to leave work earlier and spend more time on the things that I enjoy, including being with my partner and my family. I also plan on delegating more of the detail work to my assistant and will set up one meeting with her each week to accomplish this. In order to ensure that I keep more reasonable hours, I will let my staff know I am leaving early some nights, and I will ask my wife to join me downtown for a dinner date one night each week.

> Now you try it.

## Acknowledge Your Obstacles, Doubts, and Self-Sabotage

Once you have clearly written your goals, ask yourself about each goal, "What are the obstacles to accomplishing this goal? How might I sabotage myself or get in my own way of accomplishing this goal?" Write your answers in your notebook.

## Share Your Goals with Your Partner

Come together and take turns reading your lists slowly aloud to each other. First, read your list of Individual Goals, followed by your Couple Goals and conclude with your Family Goals. Do not discuss them right now. Listen carefully to each other.

Once you have shared all your goals, discuss your responses. Are your goals aligned? Talk about any surprises—not in a judgmental way, but by sharing your reactions. Talk about these lists in terms of your values and priorities and desire to have a solid partnership.

## Make a Combined Master List of One-Year Goals

Now you'll create a master list of Couple and Family goals for the coming year. Refer to the list on page 150 to use as a sample of topics you should address. Rewrite your Couple and Family goals by combining what each of you wrote. This is an opportunity to clarify your mutual goals in a common language. Make sure that the intentions, needs, and desires that each of you share are noted in your master list.

# Our Master List of Goals
## Partnering Goals

| Your Goals | Couple Goals | Family Goals | My Goals |
| --- | --- | --- | --- |
| | | | |
| | | | |
| | | | |
| | | | |
| | | | |
| | | | |
| | | | |
| | | | |

One of you may have something on your list that the other person does not. Here is an opportunity to discuss if this goal is truly acceptable to both parties. For example, a husband may wish to take a cross-country family vacation or a wife may hope to spend money on an addition to the house within the next year. They may be willing to add these to their partnership goals, or it may be that finances prohibit these goals. In this event, they have two options: One is to postpone the addition until a later time—and perhaps put it on a three-year goal list. Another is to decide on a one-year goal that is a baby step toward the bigger goal, such as going on a weekend getaway or painting several rooms in the house.

Now that you have made a joint list of goals, set your lists of Individual Goals alongside this master list.

Talk about your willingness to support each other's Individual Goals during the coming year. Share your concerns about and commitment to these Individual Goals. Talk about what will be required of each of you to support each other's goals. Referring back to a prior example, if one of you wants to exercise more regularly, the other may volunteer to watch the kids one or two evenings a week, or you may need to alter your carpooling or mealtime schedule. How can you support each other's individual needs? Some goals may be rewritten or altered in order to assure that the other partner supports a specific goal.

## Identify Your Mutual Priorities

Working together, choose which three Couple Goals you want to start working on first. (Two of them should be daily details you want to smooth out. They should be former problems or hot topics you have not thoroughly discussed since signing the Do Not Fight

Pact in Step 1. While they may seem less problematic now that you have turned them into positive goals, they potentially still require deeper discussion, which you will learn how to do in the next chapters.)

If you have a family, you will also choose one or two Family Goals from your master list. Then tell each other which two or three Individual Goals you will focus on.

Once you have mutually chosen your three partnering goals, brainstorm about each goal, one at a time, for ten minutes. Make a list for each—without judgment or edits—that includes all the possible ways you could work toward it individually and together. Write all the specific things you can accomplish as partners to make this goal a reality. Then, choose the three or four most practical steps. Circle those you could complete within the next few weeks.

Next, divide up the tasks: Who will do what and by what date? Agree to be accountable. Agree on a weekly day and time at which you will report back to each other on your progress toward the first goal. These get-togethers will now become your regular partnering meetings.

After you have a plan for this first Couple Goal, follow the same steps for your two remaining goals. Then do the same for your Individual Goals, either together or separately.

Because you'll want to make progress and feel successful, choose some goals that are less difficult and some more complex or challenging to start. For example, altering your meal planning and grocery shopping regimen may be a less complex goal than improving your sex life—although both may be on your Individual or Master Goal lists. Finding a mutually satisfying way of handling money—from paying bills to establishing savings and investment plans—is often a loaded and difficult issue, but an important one to tackle in order to have a good partnering foundation and create smoothly functioning daily details. In fact, I suggest that you select "smoother handling of finances" as your complex goal. Try to establish a series of specific action items you can accomplish in a short period of time for complex goals. For example,

One year from now, we would like to be in full agreement and well informed about all aspects of our money management. As a solid step toward this, we agree that in the next four weeks we will review our current financial status and decide on a budget to implement for this year. We agree to have Saturday-morning coffee out to review our financial progress and create new action steps to become better managers of our money. We will also obtain the names of three financial planners and make appointments with at least two of them within the next three months. We'll work with our favorite planner to understand necessary details for our financial plan going forward.

At each partnering meeting, use the following formula for brief follow-up (unless more conversation is required):

- Each of you gives a brief report on the action steps taken to accomplish the identified goal.

- Then, each of you talks through how best to 1) define your goal this week, 2) ask for help or support, 3) identify ways you might self-sabotage, and 4) describe the action steps you plan to take this week (for each goal).

After your partnering and family meetings, spend a few moments talking about what you appreciate about each other and do something fun or memorable together: popcorn and a video, a bike ride, a backyard water-balloon fight, or a build-your-own pizza dinner.

## Chapter 11

# STEP 9:

## Practice the Art of Heartfelt Listening

The Big Picture tool we'll discuss in this chapter helps you *listen for understanding when*

- you encounter a difficulty or disagreement in your communication or when you are about to work toward resolving a previously hot topic;

- one of you wants a change and the other isn't aware of the need for change;

- you want to explore a new or future Big Picture Dream together.

As you work to graduate from this 10 Step course and emerge as full-fledged Big Picture Partners, you will be taking action on the goals you clarified in Step 8. Some of these positive goals used to be unresolved issues, fights, or cold war silences between you. Because you delayed discussing them while you calmed down your relationship and worked through the initial steps of this program, these topics deserve extra-special care and attention so you can listen to each other in a new way. It is only when you have thoroughly listened to each other, when you have arrived at a clear understanding of each viewpoint, that you can work toward mutually satisfying, win/win solutions together. In this chapter, you will learn to *listen for new understanding* as you discuss goals that used to be conflicts. In the final chapter, *Step 10:* Resolve Conflict and Create New Options Together, you will learn tools to arrive at new solutions together as you work to reach your goals.

Later in this chapter, you'll read some examples of how this dialogue has been used by many other couples to listen carefully and understand their partner more fully. You'll see how this tool is useful when applied to frequent, everyday interactions, such as scheduling; hot topics or hurtful experiences, such as emotional affairs or in-law troubles; and even Big Picture Dreams you'd like to pursue. Then you'll apply the Intentional Dialogue to topics on your partnering table in the exercises at the end of this chapter.

---

**TIP:** Understanding does not require agreement. It is only when you have understanding of your two separate needs, desires, or perspectives that you can work toward creative resolution of previous conflicts, new options to smooth out your daily details, or win/win action steps to reach your Big Picture Dreams.

---

## The Intentional Dialogue Technique and Its Uses

In close relationships, people often mistakenly assume that they are listening to each other and hearing what their partner says. When a couple finds they have been facing unresolved issues for a period, they often discover through Intentional Dialogue that they are laboring under mismatched assumptions. One partner may not have truly agreed to a particular resolution or decision. That person may have been silent or grunted or rolled his or her eyes or looked at the floor. That partner may never truly have said yes or no. I always think that not saying "yes" should be taken as "no"—rather than as "maybe," "we'll see, but we need to talk more," or "no, for now."

The Intentional Dialogue is a technique for communicating about topics that are problematically difficult to hear or difficult to understand. It is a tool for listening deeply to and signaling that you have heard what another person says. This tool helps you to avoid making assumptions, so you can truly know what your partner thinks and feels. Using this tool will give each of you an opportunity to thoroughly explore and articulate all of your thoughts without being interrupted or cut off. We seldom have the opportunity to be listened to so well; in Big Picture Partnering, the Intentional Dialogue gives you both that chance.

Very often couples can't arrive at a resolution on a particular issue. But, once one person feels understood, what was once problematic is often no longer so. If there is understanding, we can work for resolution together. Often in our closest intimate relationships, we just want to be understood; we may think we need to get our partner to agree with us, but really, we just want our point of view heard and accepted, not diminished or swept under the rug. When it is your turn to assume the listener role, you may hear new things that you didn't know your partner even thought about. You may find great wisdom, some tough feedback, some deep hurts, and even great new ideas if you learn to listen.

Once you get the hang of the Intentional Dialogue, you will find that conflicts are resolved more quickly and smoothly. In addition, because your energy is not bound up in fighting or disagreements, you will unleash more energy for play, passion, fun, and even greater creativity in your relationship.

The Intentional Dialogue was originally developed in what is called Imago Relationship Therapy. Back in the early 1970s when Parent Effectiveness Training (PET) was a new and popular communication training approach, some of the foundations of the Intentional Dialogue technique were first introduced. Over the years, various educators have used the terms *paraphrasing*, *mirroring*, and *active listening* to describe aspects of this healthy approach to communication. Harville Hendrix and his colleagues compiled and combined the best of what was known about the dialogue technique and published the tools in his book *Getting The Love You Want: A Guide For Couples* (2001). It is now widely used. In my own work with couples, the Intentional Dialogue has become pivotal in helping Big Picture Partners resolve conflict.

## Learning the Intentional Dialogue Technique

When training couples in the use of the Intentional Dialogue, I initially spend about two hours reviewing and coaching them as they each play their roles as "speaker" and "listener." The couple has come to the coaching session with one or two safe but meaty topics they might like to discuss. Together they decide which of these topics to use for practice. Sometimes one partner is shy about role-playing or doesn't always follow the rules. Sometimes, one wants to edit the partner's comments.

---

**TIP:** While dialoguing in this structured way may seem unfamiliar or even silly at first, the more quickly you accept and follow the rules of the Intentional Dialogue and are willing to practice this technique, the more quickly you will learn to creatively and successfully handle stressful, difficult, or long-term issues.

---

When you first practice the Intentional Dialogue, it takes a bit of time (up to an hour for each of you to have a turn as listener and speaker). The dialogue format puts your communication into slow motion, so you can truly listen to each other and hear in a new way—without prior assumptions or misunderstandings. With a little consistent practice (three to four practice sessions), most couples become adept at applying the "mirroring" technique in three-to-five-minute mini-dialogues when they run into a minor, everyday misunderstanding.

## The Intentional Dialogue Process

There are three basic steps to the Intentional Dialogue technique: mirroring, validating, and empathizing.

### 1. Mirroring

In the Intentional Dialogue process, there is a speaker and a listener. They agree on the amount of time allotted for a dialogue. It is preferable if the speaker can talk until finished and say everything he or she wants to bring up, but this is not always feasible. In your beginning practice, try to set aside enough undisturbed time for each of you to speak as long as you need to.

The speaker gets to talk about anything that is important to him or her. Not only does the speaker get to talk as long as necessary, that partner even gets to repeat him- or herself while exploring an issue. The goal of the speaker is to talk until fully "heard" by the listener.

The role of the listener is to do just that—to listen and then to "mirror back" what the partner said. Mirroring back involves using similar, but not necessarily the same, words—much like paraphrasing. What is most important here is that the listener attempt to listen empathically, as if in the speaker's shoes. So, the listener needs to set aside personal ego in order to understand what the partner is saying, from that partner's point of view. Then the listener's task is to feed this message back to the speaker in words that show he or she has understood the partner. For example,

Susan: "I don't like it when you go to bed without saying goodnight."

Tom: "I hear you saying that you're unhappy with me when I forget to say goodnight to you before I go to bed."

Susan: "That's right."

Mirroring is different from "editorializing." An editorial comment would be, "I know just what you mean. I've felt that way myself," or "I've seen you do that when you . . ." When we editorialize or add our own comments and experience, we take the speaker out of his or her personal experience. Your task as listener is to feed back what you are hearing your partner communicate to you.

All relationships have disagreements and all people have different points of view. The Intentional Dialogue helps you get your ego out of the way so you can hear anew—so there are no assumptions or misunderstandings about what your partner is saying; so your partner can be heard for as long as he or she wishes to speak without having to think about you or your thoughts, ideas, judgments—or even your questions. All of these distract your partner from his or her deepest thoughts and feelings—thoughts and feelings your partner is trying to share with you.

So, when it is your turn to listen, listen as though you're hearing your partner for the first time. Get your ego out of the way—especially if you disagree with the version of the story or you want to correct something said or you feel wronged. Instead of focusing on your story, imagine your ego as a little character you put off to your left side. Imagine gently taking your ego by the shoulders and sitting it down next to you. Tell it firmly that its turn will come later. Right now your partner is speaking.

---

**TIP:** Your task is to listen to your partner from inside your partner's shoes, from behind his or her eyes, so you get a feeling for that person's experience—not yours. Work at mirroring thoughts and feelings with care and your partner will feel truly listened to.

---

There are not many opportunities in life to truly think aloud and hear your deepest thoughts, and then have those thoughts reflected back to you. Too often people will interrupt, think they know what you are saying, and make assumptions about where your thought is going or think of what they are going to say while you are still talking.

You can help each other with just a few simple phrases. As the listener, you might say, "tell me more" if the speaker indicates that your mirroring wasn't quite correct; or, "let me see if I've got that" when the speaker has talked for so long that you can hold no more thoughts and need to feed them back. Sometimes a little hand gesture, signaling the speaker to pause so you can mirror back what was already said also helps.

---

**TIP:** When you are the speaker, you must give clear feedback to the listener about how much you feel understood.

---

For some, to be understood 70 percent of the time is enough; others may need to be understood 93.33 percent. While the percentage of need varies, I encourage couples new at the mirroring technique to make sure they really feel like their partner is getting the essence of what they are saying. Both parties are challenged to become better at listening and clarifying their communication and their efforts will pay off in the ensuing work they do.

So, the speaker might say something like, "I know you are saying the right words, but something in the way you are repeating it back to me makes me feel like you don't quite have my full meaning. Let me try to say this a different way . . ."

I have coached couples who went back and forth like this for thirty minutes until they both had the "aha" moment when the listener had finally heard the speaker's thoughts. The difference in how you express meaning may be subtle, but when you actively listen to each other and truly hear what the other person is saying, the experience of understanding and clarity is powerful. If the speaker hasn't fully been understood yet, he or she might say, "You have the first half of what I said correct, but you forgot the second point I made. Let me say it again," or, "As I hear you repeat that, I realize it isn't what I meant at all. Let me say what I really mean." The listener's task is to pay close attention and follow the speaker's train of thought, wherever it may lead.

When the speaker finishes, when he or she feels fully understood, then the listener does two things. The first is called validating, and the second is called empathizing.

## 2. Validating

Validating is a simple statement made by the listener after mirroring what the speaker has said. It is a short statement that says, "I hear you. I understand your words. You've articulated your feelings or experience clearly." Validating lets the speaker know he or she is making sense.

Validating is one short affirming sentence. It is offered without repeating any of your partner's prior communication and without any additional comments. Continue to keep the focus on your partner as you as you say, "You are making sense." A few examples of validating statements would be as follows:

- "From everything you've told me, your experience is understandable."

- "You are making sense to me."

- "I hear you and I understand your point of view."

- "I hear you and I understand what you are saying to me."

If you are new to the Intentional Dialogue or your partner brings up a topic that is uncomfortable for you, you may feel like being silly, goofy, joking, or lighthearted to ease your discomfort. Perhaps, your partner's points may make you feel insecure, sad, angry, disappointed, controlling, or even competitive. You may want to get your side of the story into the dialogue. Wait. Focus on what your partner is saying. You will have a turn.

Remember, you need to take turns. You will get a turn to voice your opinions and your side of the story. When you are the listener, it is your job to listen to your partner. You must follow the rules and not editorialize, act silly, or be sarcastic. Such behavior will distract your partner from what he or she is trying to say. You must open your heart and listen deeply from inside the speaker's shoes. Your partner will do the same for you when it is your turn to speak.

Adding additional comments, like the following, is not part of an Intentional Dialogue:

"I've got it! Gosh, and now I understand why you always get mad and throw a fit the way you do!"

"I can really understand your experience, but don't you think if you knew how much I really loved you this wouldn't matter?"

Once again, it is important to listen to the speaker's experience nonjudgmentally, removing your ego and reactions from the dialogue. Your job is to simply say you've heard your partner and you understand.

## 3. Empathizing

Empathizing is the final step in the Intentional Dialogue process. This is a simple statement in which the listener mirrors back the feelings that have been named by the speaker or, if no feelings have been named, the feelings the listener senses are unspoken. If the listener is off base, the dialogue may segue back into another little round of mirroring until there is again full understanding. Here are two examples of empathizing. The first example shows simple clarity:

Listener: "Everything you are saying makes sense, and I can hear just how frustrated and angry you are, how it even makes you want to give up."

Speaker: "Yes! That's exactly how I've been feeling."

In the second example, the speaker clarifies his or her feelings:

Listener: "Gee, honey, from everything you are saying, I get it. I can imagine that you must be feeling very sad and distant from me as a result."

Speaker: "Actually, I no longer feel sad about it. I've gotten to the point at which your lack of communicating just makes me downright mad. I don't deserve to be treated this way. Just so I'm being clear—I'm not going to throw a tantrum anymore even though I'm mad. And, I am only going to do my part in the communicating process. Otherwise, we won't grow together."

Listener: "Let me see if I've got that. You're not really sad. You've become resolved. You are really angry, but you are not going to yell about it anymore. You are clear. You're not going to take my passivity or fear or stubbornness as your problem anymore. You want me to know that either I communicate or we won't have the kind of relationship we both say we want. Did I get that right?"

Speaker: "You bet! That's exactly what I'm saying!"

Listener: "That's exactly what you mean. Is there more?"

Speaker: "No. I feel finished."

Listener again validates: "Once again, you make even more sense and I hear you."

Listener again empathizes: "And you made it clear you are feeling mad and resolute."

Speaker: "That's for sure!"

In the best scenario, the partners would then exchange roles and go through the entire process again to mirror, validate, and empathize with the other person. If immediate role reversal is not possible, they agree to give the previous listener a turn to be the speaker within two days. By doing so they agree not to discuss the topic until the dialogue is complete.

## Using the Intentional Dialogue in Your Partnership

In the initial stages of practicing the Intentional Dialogue, plan to use this technique about once each week for about a month as you apply it to problems you turned into positive goals. In the beginning, set aside an hour for each dialogue so you each get a half-hour as listener and speaker.

Eventually you will mirror, validate, and empathize as a frequent part of your everyday communication. When you reach that point, three situations will need a formal Intentional Dialogue:

### 1. One Partner Requests a Dialogue

It doesn't matter why. The immediate Big Picture response is, "Okay, when shall we schedule a time? I'll be there." No questions asked. No hemming and hawing. If an issue is important to one of you, it is important to the partnership. (Remember *Step 5:* Address Any Issue Together—Whether It's Yours, Mine, or Ours.)

### 2. A Stressful or Problematic Issue Arises That Causes Fighting

This situation will be more easily resolved if you use the Intentional Dialogue the minute you sense a fight beginning. If you are too angry or heated, take a time-out or cool down first. Then agree to use the dialogue when you are both ready to listen.

## 3. An Exciting Opportunity Arises

When you have exciting life-transition goals, big events, or creative projects you are planning, Intentional Dialogue may help you speed the positive change. Sharing goals and ideas becomes smooth and safe. You can listen to each other calmly.

Some couples use the dialogue frequently on seemingly mundane issues, but when they do, it keeps their relationship flowing more smoothly. Arnold and Beth are such an example. They frequently use the mirroring portion of the Intentional Dialogue technique around scheduling activities for themselves and their four young children. Without it, they run into many snafus due to not listening carefully enough to each other, and their children frequently missed an after school event or dinner with the family! They stop for five minutes while Arnold repeats back, "Okay, so I'm to pick up Annie at school tonight at 4:00 p.m., bring her home for supper, then I'll take Annie and Joey to hockey practice while you, Sarah, and the baby go grocery shopping. Is that right?" By mirroring back what his wife has said about the schedule, he clarifies for both of them that he's heard Beth clearly and everyone will get to their correct destination on time!

Beth frequently uses the same technique when she needs to know Arnold's inconsistent travel schedule or when he will be at the office on weekends. Frequent mirroring saves them lots of time and misunderstanding in this very active family.

The Intentional Dialogue is also useful when approaching hot or hurtful topics. It was a pivotal tool for the following two couples as they grappled with the hurt and anger of an emotional affair that could have become explosive and a prickly mother-in-law relationship that could have deteriorated into withdrawal.

Sam and Jessica were trying to rebuild their relationship after an emotional affair. Jessica was feeling unloved by Sam due to his lack of attention. The advances of another man, while she was out with girlfriends one night, led to a series of text, e-mail, and telephone encounters. Physical monogamy was not breached, and the infatuation quickly resolved itself, as both Jessica and the other man were married with kids. When Jessica decided she needed to be open with Sam about her flirtation if she was going to work on her marriage, Sam was deeply hurt, angry, and self-protective. They found it difficult to talk without exploding or blaming on either side. After a number of blow ups, the couple agreed to work on the many issues underlying this threat to their connection. Because they loved each other and wanted to make their relationship better and "affair-proof," Sam and Jessica worked hard to become better partners. The Intentional Dialogue became a powerful tool for initially talking through their hurtful and heated emotions regarding the betrayal and the problems that led up to this event. Then they applied the dialogue to the list of issues that had gone under the rug and made them feel disconnected. As they did so, their relationship became more solid and satisfying for both of them.

The Intentional Dialogue was also significant in Karen and Matt's partnership as they tackled a variety of problems. Married for seven years, one topic that was particularly thorny for Karen was her relationship with Matt's mom whom Karen felt was overbearing. Matt could see that his mom was always imparting advice—making it clear that she knew how to please Matt and Karen did not. Growing up, Matt had learned to tune out his mother's constant meddling. Because he loved both women, he felt helpless not knowing what to do or how to help Karen—or how to stop his mom.

Karen felt abandoned by Matt's passivity in the matter and especially at his withdrawal from any conversation about his mother or her impact on their relationship as a couple. When they learned to listen using the Intentional Dialogue, Karen heard that Matt did understand her quandary. While giving Karen his attention and listening to her frustrations, Matt also had a turn to clarify that he was not taking his mother's side but rather, he did not know what to do. This dialogue helped them understand each other's position and gave them an opportunity to express empathy. Neither Karen nor Matt wanted his mom to come between them; nor did they want to cut off this important relationship, frustrating as it sometimes was. Dialogue led to feeling more connected—like allies—when they visited Matt's parents even though his mother's behavior did not change.

The Intentional Dialogue can also help you to discuss the dreams and bigger goals you want to pursue as a couple. For example, Vicki and Todd agreed she would go back to graduate school in a year or two. Dialogues helped them to talk through the many alterations they needed to make in their finances, schedules, work life, and even how they managed their chores when Vicki would be going to classes some nights and on weekends.

Steve and Sharon found similar benefits as they discussed their dream of purchasing a sailboat in their later years and spending several months of the year sailing along the southern coast. This was a long-term plan they slowly implemented, working out many details including finances, relationships with two college-aged daughters, managing a home in the

Midwest, continuing Steve's real estate company, and downsizing Sharon's position in a small law firm from full time to part time.

Listening for understanding for each of these couples brought up many concerns and initiated many new ideas about how to pursue their dreams.

The Intentional Dialogue takes time and practice to master, but as you can see in the examples above, the benefits are great. In the exercises that follow, we'll break it down into some doable steps. First, you will become acquainted with the Intentional Dialogue and its format. Next, you will practice informally. Then, you will practice formally as you apply it to some of your goals that were former unresolved issues or problems between you.

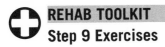

## REHAB TOOLKIT
## Step 9 Exercises

### *Become Acquainted with the Intentional Dialogue Technique*

Come together and discuss your understanding of the three-step Intentional Dialogue process: mirroring, validating, and empathizing. Review the rules for using the dialogue and discuss what you each think it means to be an active listener. Next, as you go about your lives, notice the conversations you overhear and participate in when the Intentional Dialogue might be helpful.

### Practice Informal "Mirroring"

In everyday interactions, start to practice and play with mirroring—but not so much that it becomes annoying. Just once in awhile start to adopt the mirroring language: "Just making sure, hon. You want me to put the kids to bed tonight, right?" Start to use it in conversations.

### Practice Formally

Schedule two times during one week to practice the Intentional Dialogue with each other. Set aside at least one uninterrupted hour for each practice session.

In Step 8, you chose one or two goals to achieve together that used to be problematic daily details. Choose one goal to discuss during this practice session. You have not discussed the underlying differences since you signed the Do Not Fight Pact in Step 1. While the differences may no longer be problematic, use the Intentional Dialogue carefully as you venture into sharing why this goal is important to you, what is or is not working for you, and the changes you would prefer in managing this daily detail going forward.

Decide who will be the first speaker. The speaker will have thirty minutes to talk while the listener practices mirroring, validating, and empathizing. Then you will switch roles. Due to the time limit, you may not complete a full Intentional Dialogue. That is fine; this time is mainly for practice.

If you feel you have run out of things to say, still practice for the entire thirty minutes. You can do these four things to expand on your thoughts:

- Repeat your points using more examples and new words.

- Go deeper—talk about how unresolved issues or daily details make you feel.

- Make sure you talk about how you would like your relationship to be if these things were no longer problems.

- Tell your partner what other interests you'd like to pursue if the daily details flowed like clockwork.

As you practice the Intentional Dialogue, pause and start over if any of these things happen:

- You lose your train of thought as the speaker or forget where you are in the Intentional Dialogue process.

- Your ego gets in the way or you get angry as the listener. If this happens, pause and note what you are feeling. Don't act inappropriately or say anything. Breathe, and remember you will have a turn to speak. When you are ready, return to active listening.

- You find yourself editing the speaker by adding your own comments, thoughts, or interpretations—rather than mirroring, validating, and empathizing.

After each practice session, do not debrief. Allow yourselves to absorb what you have shared. Two or three days later, do another Intentional Dialogue during which you discuss the same issues raised in the last session. The partner who went second last time will go first this time.

Continue to use this valuable tool in the years ahead. Apply the longer Intentional Dialogue formally as you work to resolve problems and achieve your bigger goals together. Use mirroring for understanding more informally when an issue comes up that is easily clarified. Put the topic, assumption, or misunderstanding on your partnering table; listen and mirror for understanding.

## Chapter 12

# STEP 10:
## Resolve Conflict and Create New Options Together

You may have picked up this book because you were in trouble, your relationship had gone stale, or you wanted to get partnering right this time. You've worked hard to practice each of the steps. Big Picture Partnering is meant to move you from reactivity to proactivity, from problems to creative problem solving together. And, you each know how you'd like to handle many situations if you are on your own.

During this final chapter of *Romance Rehab*, you'll practice applying **Step 10: Resolve Conflict and Create New Options Together** to the goals you developed in Step 8, as well as to the any conflicts that existed when you began reading this book. Together you will

- invent new options through brainstorming and building on each other's ideas;

- discuss which ideas are mutually satisfying;

- choose solutions that are win/wins for both of you;

- close the loop and agree on applying win/win solutions;

- experiment and explore as you try your new options;

- reevaluate and refine action steps as you achieve your goal.

The options you create are the way to resolve differences or problems. They will become your Big Picture path to reach goals and realize dreams together.

## Discovering New Options

By now, you are familiar with the concepts of Your World, My World, and Our World, and you know that nothing goes into Our World until it is fully agreed upon and has become a win/win for both of you. In practice, however, many couples hit a stumbling block when they bring their individual suggestions to the table for discussion or problem solving. Some partners may fail to see that there are other possible alternatives to their proposed solution, or they may naively imagine that their partner will be enthusiastic about a suggestion, only to be crestfallen when the other person says, "I'm sorry honey, but I don't like that idea."

Tim and Sophie became stuck during their discussions. They were in full agreement about their one-year goals, but they had different ideas about how to achieve them.

Tim reflected,

> Way back in the beginning of setting our one-year goals, we both wanted to get into better shape within about six months. I had gained about thirty extra pounds and wanted to take that off. Sophie hadn't been exercising, except for chasing after our two-year-old, and we wanted to find some things to do together, because our time is limited. I was doing a lot of reading about diets and brought up an easy but healthy diet, which I was excited about. Sophie quickly agreed to join in, and we have been doing the diet for three months now. I've lost a lot of weight and feel much better. It's easy with both of us eating the same way.

Sophie added,

> I was glad to do the diet. Not that I needed to lose a lot of weight, but I wanted to regulate my eating for a while and it seemed a good idea to do this together. But then, when it came to the exercise part—Tim is a fanatic! He loves to run and lift weights. I used to run, too, and he kept saying, "Just come running with me. It will be fun. We can do it together!"

Tim agreed,

Yeah, I really tried to twist Sophie's arm and forgot to partner. I thought she should enjoy doing it, because she used to like to run and I enjoy it. Finally, I paid attention enough to hear her trying to tell me how tired she was after taking care of the baby and how she no longer enjoyed running.

Sophie explained,

Tim finally did hear me, but then we needed some help to figure out where to go from there so we could agree on the kind of exercise approach we both wanted.

Tim and Sophie were successful in partnering on a diet because they both agreed on a method. Their different thoughts about an exercise regimen, however, led to many arguments between them. For a time, Tim was sure his idea should be adopted, and Sophie simply voiced all the reasons why this wouldn't work for her. She wanted Tim to understand her point of view.

Three things were missing from Tim and Sophie's conversations: First, in trying to jump to a solution too quickly, Tim and Sophie were not engaging in dialogue and not actively listening to each other's needs. Second, Tim thought Sophie should simply accept an exercise form that worked for him, forgetting that Big Picture Partnering requires a win/win decision. Third, although Sophie wanted Tim to fully understand her objections to his idea, she didn't offer any new ideas that would have promoted a dialogue toward agreement.

As you explore the lessons in this chapter, let's also consider another couple that applied *Step 10: Resolve Conflict and Create New Options Together* to their problems. Rachel and Levi had parenting problems that were tearing them apart. Married for fifteen years, Rachel and Levi had two sons. Their relationship seemed pretty satisfactory until their second child came along. Aaron, the older son, was eleven. He was a good kid, fairly easygoing and quieter than seven-year-old Josh. Josh was a handful for the entire family due to frequent angry or emotional outbursts that his mother managed but that triggered his father's rage and dictatorial discipline and that caused his older brother to withdraw. These parents worked full time, and evenings at home had deteriorated into chaos until Rachel and Levi could barely connect on anything. Their frustration was aimed at each other. Rachel felt Levi was acting just as childish and out-of-control as their son. She was concerned that the older son was being ignored. She also felt that Josh needed some help to manage his emotions, but he would not get it as long as Levi continued to blame her for not being able to discipline their son and stop his tantrums.

On the verge of divorce, this couple finally reached for some help and agreed to work through the 10 Steps of Big Picture Partnering. Theirs was not a smooth, uphill road, but they persisted because they still loved each other, and divorce would be just as difficult as trying to work things out.

These partnerships were not finding ways to come together. Both Tim and Sophie and Rachel and Levi had to let go of their old notions of how things should be in order to invent new options. They often became stuck by limiting their solutions to only one or two that were obvious at the time. Remember, a duel to the death is an option. So is a shouting match. What is important about discovering new solutions is that they must be mutually desired, mutually chosen, and mutually beneficial. You may find that getting stuck on one idea happens in your relationship. Then what? You might let the topic drop. It might go unresolved. Then, one of you may bring it up again, and the same old unworkable solutions are rehashed, ending with the same old stalemate. Like Tim and Sophie, and many other couples, you may forget to think creatively when you're in a stalemate situation. Like Rachel and Levi, you may blame each other and think the only solution is for the other person to change. Let's see how learning to partner and creating new options worked for each of them. It can work for you.

## Inventing New Options Gets You out of a Rut

While their relationship was not in trouble, both Tim and Sophie wanted to live long, healthy lives and bring good nutrition and consistent exercise into their lifestyle. They valued doing it together to strengthen their partnership and to have active time together.

Tim and Sophie were stuck on how to arrive at a mutually satisfying exercise program they could consistently share.

They had their goal. Applying Step 10 of the process, Tim and Sophie laid out their individual ideas. Tim's choice was for he and Sophie to go running together. Sophie responded,

> I'm not interested in running or training for a race like you are, but I do like to walk, and if you would consider compromising, I'd do some brisk walking with you three times a week after dinner.

## ✚ REHAB TOOLKIT
## Steps to Brainstorming

You've heard the term *brainstorming* many times before. You may have used this technique at work or at community meetings. Let's review the process so you can use it to help you become more imaginative:

- Set a time limit. You might start with five minutes.

- Have a sheet of paper on which one of you records all the ideas you are going to throw on the table during those five minutes.

- Remember that the ideas are potential responses to the problem or goal you are addressing at the time.

- Allow the ideas to be as wild and crazy or as practical as you wish.

- Do not censor any ideas. Simply keep the ball rolling while you brainstorm nonstop for five minutes.

- If you fall silent before the five minutes are up, simply wait quietly. You or your partner may think of another idea in time!

- Apply your list of ideas to the Map It Out exercise on page 174 and to the activities at the end of this week.

---

Brisk walking was now on the table; however, Tim wasn't buying into it. At this point, Tim and Sophie were encouraged to keep these individual options on the table, and to come up with at least three totally different ideas that pleased them both. They slowly began to play with ideas together. Tim said,

> I'm wondering if we don't both need to do something totally new. When I really listen to Sophie and mirror back what she is saying, I learn more details about what she is saying. Sophie is telling me that she wants an exercise that's 1) challenging, but 2) not harsh, and 3) fits into our odd schedules. I also like a challenge, and I can also work with her to find something not too harsh for her and an exercise that fits into our schedules—so all of her needs get met, and I am happy too.

As they talked together, they invented three new options: joining a regular evening Pilates class, purchasing exercise equipment for a home gym, and taking private yoga classes. In addition to listening and mirroring, they tried the Steps to Brainstorming exercise you'll find on pages 173 and the Map It Out exercise you'll find below. Sophie remarked,

> Mapping out our options on paper was fun. I think we were both surprised at how difficult it was to come up with three solutions we both agreed on, but after brainstorming at least ten ideas, we narrowed down our top choices to the three we could both enjoy. Then we started to get excited about the new alternatives.

Said Tim,

> We talked about each idea, and the private yoga instruction really excited both of us. Now we love yoga, and we can schedule the lessons any time of the day or evening.

Sophie added,

> Both of us love the new challenge. We can be doing the very same yoga movement, but I can go at my own pace and so can Tim. It's perfect for us.

## ✚ REHAB TOOLKIT
## Map It Out

You might try to map your newly interconnected ideas as you converse, in order to gain a visual picture of how your ideas relate to and enhance each other's. Draw two circles on your partnering table. In one circle, write your solution to the problem. In the other circle, write your partner's solution to the problem.

Now write the many ideas you have brainstormed in a list on the side of your table. Draw three more circles in the table and talk about which brainstormed ideas are mutually satisfying, win/win solutions to your goal or problem. As you find these win/win options, highlight them and discuss how you will practice implementing them in the coming days or weeks.

This exercise will help you come together, rather than focus on ways you are dissimilar. It will help you to generate a creative flow of ideas that both of you can enthusiastically endorse.

## Inventing New Options May Save Your Sanity

Rachel and Levi's situation was much more tenuous. They had to work hard to practice the earlier partnering steps and calm their relationship down before they could apply Step 10. Gradually they stopped sniping and snarling at each other and behaved in a more adult manner. As they did so, they created pockets of time to talk and managed to have less chaotic dinners and bedtimes—enough so they stayed connected as a couple and as a family.

Then they dialogued about many things and especially their different thoughts on Josh's outbursts and how to parent him. As they realized they needed to come up with new solutions to their disagreements instead of stubbornly holding their private positions, Rachel and Levi began to learn to invent new options together.

They applied these new options to their son's outbursts and to their reaction to his outbursts. Levi's old stance was to yell at Rachel and tell her to make Josh behave. Then he would sulk all night, remaining disconnected from his wife even if Josh had quieted down. Rachel's old response was to yell back and take Josh to his room and hold him tightly until he had stopped flailing and fighting back and then cried and calmed down enough to talk to her. This sometimes took more than an hour.

As they tried the Steps to Brainstorming exercise on page 173, Levi and Rachel came up with these options: 1) They could take Josh to a therapist to see what was wrong and get outside help; 2) one parent could handle the situation at any one time while the other left the room and did not interfere; or 3) they could tell Josh that his outbursts were no longer OK. If he was frustrated, it was OK to feel that way, but he'd have to go to his room until he felt calmer. Then he could rejoin the family. Josh could also be given two choices of activities or foods to select from. This idea came up because Josh seemed to melt down whenever he wanted something but was not given a choice in the matter. Brainstorming also raised a discussion of how Levi was going to behave differently than in the past since he had been demonstrating behavior similar to Josh's behavior. They agreed that if they wanted Josh to change, Levi would also have to change.

Out of this list of new options, Rachel and Levi agreed to not interfere with each other's parenting decisions until they obtained a family therapist's professional opinion on how to proceed. The therapist applauded their efforts at brainstorming, and confirmed that Josh's issues were behavioral and changeable with more structure in the family life. Then she encouraged this couple find the win/wins they could implement to help their son.

Feeling buoyed with renewed optimism, Rachel and Levi utilized the Map It Out exercise on page 174 to help them arrive at mutually satisfying next steps they could agree on. They quickly chose to give Josh choices and also to send him to his room to manage his feelings when he became upset. They both agreed to be loving but firm rather than blaming, judgmental, or dictatorial with Josh. Together—as a united front—they presented these new conditions to Josh. They did so in a matter-of-fact and calm manner. Within two weeks of consistent practice, Josh's behavior became more appropriate. When he did experience a meltdown and was sent to his room, he accepted the ground rules and learned to comfort himself until he was ready to come out and talk or rejoin family activities.

In this calmer atmosphere, Rachel and Levi continued to reconnect and resolve other issues on their partnering table. They also found ways to provide their eleven-year-old with more attention that had previously gone only to Josh. Aaron began to come out of his shell. The entire family life improved as Josh gradually learned to manage his emotions and his parent's partnership was strengthened. The threat of divorce disappeared.

Just like Tim and Sophie or Rachel and Levi, your communication toward satisfying solutions may become stuck. Shifting your responses to build on each other's ideas is an approach you will want to add to your toolkit.

## Build on Each Other's Ideas

Another positive behavior to replace your old negative interactions is to build on each other's ideas rather than ignore or disagree. For example, when your partner shares an idea or a thought, once you have listened thoroughly, respond by saying,

> "Let me build on that idea." Or, "Would it be all right if I built on that idea?"

> "Let me add to that thought." Or, "Would it be all right if I added to that thought?"

As you practice this strategy, you will experience the building-block effect of reciprocal ideas being exchanged. You will create a network of interlocking ideas, rather than ideas that are conflicting, disjointed, or disconnected.

The following are additional phrases that you can use to build on each other's ideas or thoughts (of course, feel free to come up with your own as well.):

- "I can see that if (refer to what your partner has just shared), then . . ."

- "I can imagine that if we (refer to what your partner has just said), then . . ."

- "I am wondering if we also . . ."

- "I'd like to explore that option some more and add . . ."

- "What if we did what you suggest and then also experimented with . . ."

At first you may want to mimic and play, just to practice, until you each find the phrases that feel right to you. The aim is to continue to come together, build on each other's ideas, and intensify the creative flow of ideas.

## Choose Win/Wins and Close the Loop

Here's how the process goes: You identified your mutual goal and listened for understanding. Now, following the Map It Out exercise on page 174, invent new ideas together. They may be playfully wild and crazy just to get you started. Stretch to add many ideas that are realistic or doable. Brainstorm and build on each other's ideas as you come up with new options. Discuss which concepts are mutually agreeable. Sometimes aspects of two or three suggestions form the right solution. That's OK. Then *close the loop*. This means that together you identify the option or options that are mutually satisfying. If more than one option is a win/win, choose your favorite to practice as a solution to your former problem. Then discuss what each of you will to do, when and how you will each follow through as you try this newly invented solution to resolve a former problem and reach your desired goal. Closing the loop means coming to agreement and developing a timetable to experiment. After you have tried your new solution for a time, you will come back and evaluate how they are going, then refine your action steps.

## Experiment and Explore as You Try Your New Options

Frequent experimenting with new ideas or options and exploring to see if you like or enjoy something new can be fun. It also makes you resilient, ready for changes that come your way, and ready to pivot or change course because you become familiar with change and how to navigate through it. Experimenting and exploring also brings a little spice to life. If we wear something flashy, learn a new dance move, eat unique foods, or approach our partner with a fresh perspective, new doors can open. Experimenting and exploring in little ways makes us ready for bigger considerations. It makes us ready for anything big we might like to change or bring into our lives. Some examples of this type of change are planning for a new baby, a new pet, a new job, a move to a new city, a new house, attending a different church or synagogue, a new way to handle your finances or friendships, and so on.

Let's look at Paul and Maude's situation: They were focused on a Partnering Goal. As Paul explained it,

> We both thought we wanted to live in the suburbs about ten years ago, when we had three little kids. We considered this even though we were both raised in a medium-sized city.

Said Maude,

> Yeah, we should have found a way to check out suburban living without having to uproot ourselves and the kids, but I guess that was part of our experiment— to figure out where and how we all wanted to live.

Paul remarked,

> It was a disruptive experiment, but now we all know. We sold our great old house and bought a big rambler about thirty-five minutes from downtown. We only lived there two years, because we just missed the city too much. We all had such strong ties to our old friends and neighbors, the city shops and cultural centers. We found ourselves constantly driving into town!

Maude added,

> Finally, we just gave up and moved back to the city and into a different house in our old neighborhood. At least we know where we want to be, and everyone got the suburb fantasy out of their systems.

## The Path to Satisfaction May Be Experimental

Just like Maude and Paul who were focusing on Partnering Goals, you might try changing some of your weekly routines or daily habits to see how it feels, to spice things up, to get you out of ruts. Think about your goals and how rigidly you might hold to a specific vision of how you'd like things to turn out. Such a vision might lead to fulfillment, but it could also hinder you from seeing other possibilities—and prevent you from experimenting and exploring with your partner. Why not become more experimental and explore your goals together until you "feel your way" toward what is right for the two of you? You can still envision what you'd like, but as you feel your way toward your goals, your choices become organic to both of you. Let me further describe what I mean by choices evolving organically. It is the difference between following a goal created only in your head versus following a vision that satisfies both head and heart, a vision that develops with experience.

One reason change takes time is that we need time to learn from our experimentation—to sense whether we have become enriched by our experiences. I am not suggesting that you engage in experiments that cause you to stray from your goals. I am referring to the experiment and exploration that lead you to self-knowledge about what gives you pleasure, what suits you, what is truly satisfying. Sometimes experimentation and exploration open new doors, especially when you include other people's feedback, perspectives, thoughts, and experience.

As you apply your newly invented options, you can stretch your creativity even further by consciously experimenting and exploring, individually and together.

## Reevaluate and Refine Your Action Steps

In Big Picture Partnering, the process of defining and reaching your goals is an ongoing, cyclical one. As you funnel your differences, disagreements, desires, and dreams into Individual, Couple, and Family goals, and invent new ways of accomplishing these goals together, your connection will stay strong and your relationship will remain vital.

Once you have experimented and explored, joine together at a scheduled time—in a regular talking time, over coffee, on a dinner date, or in a family meeting—and share how far you've come. This is the time to evaluate together what things are working and which things you'd like to refine as you work toward your goal or goals. If problems have arisen, reach into your toolkit and listen for understanding using the Intentional Dialogue. Once you understand, then you naturally circle back into inventing new options, choosing new win/win solutions, and applying them to your goals. This is how you reevaluate, refine, and eventually achieve your goals together.

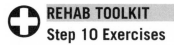

## REHAB TOOLKIT
## Step 10 Exercises

### *Using Each Other's Ideas as Building Blocks*

Individually, practice using the phrases on page 177 in all of your communications this week. Do this playfully at first if the suggested phrases feel awkward. Gradually, the process will become more natural as you find your own favorite phrases.

Notice if there is a difference in your conversations as you practice building creatively on each other's ideas. Share your observations with your partner when you come together to invent new options.

### Practice Generating New Options

This week, as you work on your partnership goals, practice creating new options with your partner. Refer back to your list of goals. Choose one or two daily details that were previously problematic to focus on first in these exercises. Your goal is to invent new solutions together so that the daily details are smoothed and no longer problematic. As you become adept at resolving daily details, then apply the exercise to a Big Picture Dream.

Here's a more detailed look at how this process might work. Have a number of sheets of loose paper handy. Start by writing the goal or problem you are trying to resolve on a sheet of paper both of you can look at as you work together. Be sure to identify the previous problem—or newly stated positive goal—in terms that you both understand. For example, Dan and Sue, a couple in a Big Picture workshop, stated their problem as follows:

> We need to refurbish our current kitchen and makes some updates. Dan would run out and simply purchase new appliances in a day and have them installed, whereas Sue loves to do research and find out everything she can about the best possible range and different vents, types of flooring, and so on. This takes her months. We want to use this process of coming up with new options to make decisions about our kitchen update. We want to complete the process within one month from today.

Refer to the Map It Out exercise on page 174 as needed.

Under your stated goal, draw your Big Picture universe with Individual and Our World circles. Use one whole sheet of paper for drawing your partnering table. Draw two circles in the partnering table. Write your solution to the problem/goal in one circle and write your partner's in the other. These are options *A* and *B*.

Returning to Sue and Dan,

- In Circle *A*, Sue wrote that she preferred a particular brand of range that was top of the line and very expensive. She knew she and Dan would need to figure out their budget to make this $5,000 purchase. She wondered if that dollar amount would allow her to also have the other appliances and the tile flooring she would like to have installed.

- In Circle *B*, Dan said he had researched the budget and felt they could afford about $6,000 total for the updates. He would rather spend a lesser amount on a number of good appliances and have enough left over for a tile floor.

Now you each write your first choice in your circles. Stop and discuss what each of you usually does at this point that may contribute to a stalemate or prevent the conversation from moving toward agreement. Talk about what you each have to let go of in order to come together to find mutually satisfying options.

Then, together, brainstorm a list of six to ten other possibilities (refer to the Steps to Brainstorming toolkit on page 173. Some ideas may be practical; some may be wild and crazy. Write all of these ideas on a separate sheet of paper.

## Discuss Which Inventions Are Mutually Satisfying

Now discuss each new idea and identify those that best satisfy both your needs. If we could observe Sue and Dan, you'd hear them agreeing that $6,000 was a pretty decent budget assessment. Sue said she really did know that the $5,000 range was extravagant. She just wanted a better range because they loved to cook together, and they liked to entertain. Dan said he could understand but asked if Sue would be willing to research together good but less expensive appliances. They put this approach on their brainstorming list along with the $6,000 budget. They listed stores and Web sites they could research for high-end products with low-end prices. Within fifteen minutes, Sue and Dan had multiple options and simply needed to research them. They needed to experiment and explore. They divided the research and agreed to meet back at the dining room table within one week to continue working toward a mutually satisfying solution to their kitchen update. Keeping to a timetable was meant to slow Tim down and speed Sue up! They agreed to stick with the one-month timetable they had chosen.

## Choose Solutions That Are Win/Wins for Both of You

Now it is your turn. Look over your list and draw three, four, or five circles floating outside the Our World circle for options *C*, *D*, and *E*.

Once you have dialogued, put the top ideas into these circles. Continue talking and listening to each other in order to agree on the option you would most like to try out together. This option goes into the Our World circle.

## Close the Loop and Agree on Applying the Win/Win Solutions

Experiment with this option in the coming weeks for an agreed-upon length of time to determine if it truly helps you meet your goals. (Remember, you can always choose another option to try out later if the first one proves unsatisfying.) Continue to use this method whenever you are stuck in making progress toward mutual goals.

Let me give a final note on Sue and Dan's kitchen. They proudly came back to the Big Picture workshop two weeks after their first brainstorming session. Each had spent a few hours researching tiles and appliances. Sue had agreed to give Dan the lead on tile and she took the lead on appliances, finding an excellent second choice for a range she would love. Dan found some tile options and out of the six samples he brought home, they chose their favorite together once they ran the costs and decided that any of the tile samples would fit this need. Once the main choices for tile and range were completed, Sue and Dan had $2,200 remaining in their budget for the other appliances and gadgets. They smoothly made these choices. Sue agreed to place all the orders and prepare for deliveries and Dan called their repairperson, plumber, and electrician. The kitchen was fully installed within one week of their desired due date. They planned a dinner party with close friends to celebrate!

# Continue Your Big Picture Adventure

You have worked together consistently and creatively to strengthen your partnership. You have experienced the winning combination of the 10 Steps and your mutual creativity. Now you know you can create most of what you want at every age and stage of your lives. This is the beginning of a lifelong process.

As we conclude this program, you will create a partnering date book that will help you continue working toward your Big Picture Goals—from the satisfying daily details to the juicy big dreams. Customize your date book together as you continue to create the partnership and life of your dreams.

## Where Do We Go from Here?

You may be asking the question, "Where do we go from here? We still have more goals on our one-year lists that we want to accomplish." You have daily details, maybe a few unresolved issues, and you may even be thinking about some future projects or dreams. Throughout the past 10 Steps, you have spent time regularly talking and actively listening to each other. You have completed many exercises individually and then come together, writing your goals and taking action steps to accomplish them. This is the process you will continue. To do this you will,

- regularly repeat the exercises in Steps 8–10 as you continue to balance your Individual, Partnership, and Family goals, as well as set new targets;

- create a Big Picture date book to reinforce the 10 Steps and to continue working on your goals.

## The Date Book

The aim of the date book is to make the *Romance Rehab* process continuous and ongoing throughout your lives. It is an agreement you make together to continue building your Big Picture. If you have not yet finished smoothing your daily details or settling unresolved issues, continue to make these your priority. Then, gradually, your date book can help you work toward those bigger goals and future dreams.

Perhaps your date book will include plans for how you want to live when the kids are grown and away from home. Maybe it will include a schedule of dialogue about where you want to go for that long-awaited vacation or sabbatical you have talked about for so long. Maybe you'll need to schedule talking times to discuss major career changes, starting a family, remodeling your home, or ways to socialize with your neighbors or contribute to your church or community. Whatever your vision might be, it is important to set new goals regularly in your life together. Your Big Picture Partnering date book will help you do so.

## Will Your Date Book Resemble Reba and Warren's?

Reba and Warren are a couple in their late forties. They have no children and are both professionals with active careers. When Warren and Reba sat down to create their date book, they began by assessing how far they'd come since they began using the partnering approach.

Warren recalled,

There is no question, we are definitely committed to talking regularly—that is a given. It has improved our connection. Talking and making sure we do nice things for each other—both are a must! We've already become adept at getting these into our daily and weekly schedules.

Our household routines—errands and grocery shopping, yard and auto upkeep, and taking turns cooking each night—have gone more smoothly. These used to be such a pain! We spent more time fighting about these things—and now, we just do them and spend time on our art projects or outdoor sports instead.

As they continued to share their experiences, Reba and Warren noted a few daily details that were still on their goal lists. One important area was financial planning. Warren said,

> We've agreed to continue getting our finances under control in the next three to six months, especially as it will impact the long-range planning we want to do. We're agreeing to meet every other week for an hour to discuss action steps, look at the bills, consolidate our expenses, and plan ways to save money for the future.

Reba noted,

> Our desire is to have completed our daily details goals six months from now so that those aspects of our lives are no-brainers. Then our goal is to look at what we'd like to create for fun in the coming ten to fifteen years when we'll have more fun time and more free time.

Reba and Warren went on to describe the future goals they had established. Warren explained,

> At this stage, we want to give back to the world. In evaluating our values and priorities, we got clear—we have no kids, we have enough money, and we still have lots of energy and half our lives left to live. We started to discuss and reevaluate how to integrate giving something back to humanity. Our discussions are new and our brainstorming list includes everything from volunteering to build Habitat for Humanity houses to joining the Red Cross Disaster Relief Teams, either nationally or internationally. Our goal is to come up with activities we can do each year that may eventually become our next "career" together.

Reba and Warren then highlighted a list of topics to put in their date book. Over the next few months, they would discuss one or two of these topics at each partnering meeting. As you'll note, most of these topics have to do with carving out more free time and balancing home and work . . . and then there's that one final item:

- Have a date night out, just the two of us, every other week
- Socialize with mutual friends, every other week

- Create more alone time

- Go to the health club three times a week (Reba)

- Run most mornings before work (Warren)

- Have dinner together most nights/coordinate so work meetings don't take precedence

- Attend monthly book club (Reba)

- Play squash or golf three to four times a month (Warren)

- Spice up our sex life!

Reba and Warren laughed as they were reminded of how much they still needed to keep balancing their daily details.

Reba concluded,

Let's just say we are still in the brainstorming stage, until we come up with a few more options that we are ready to try. Since these are six-to-twelve-month goals, we have a little time to rework how we do all of this together.

## Josh and Amanda's Date Book: A Family Affair

Josh and Amanda are in their mid-thirties with two children and a baby on the way. Erin is eight years old and Hannah is five. Here are Josh and Amanda's daily details goals, which they'll list in their partnering date book. Note how these issues highlight their stage in life and how their children are included in the scheduling.

- Stick to our regular talking times

- Figure out how Amanda can quit work and stay home once the baby comes

- Work together better as parents

- Keep practicing the Intentional Dialogue, so it becomes second nature and we don't have to schedule such long talks

- Put lovemaking on our future list—after the baby comes

- Continue our Sunday afternoon family meetings

- Reevaluate how we want our parents involved once the baby arrives

And now listen in as Amanda and Josh discuss how they came up with their list. Amanda explained,

> We're pretty good at talking, but it takes some effort to stick to our schedule. We both feel better when we stick to the regularly scheduled talking times. The girls notice the difference, too. We're more patient with each other and with them after we've had our talks—so they're calmer.
>
> Also, we want to work harder on the basics, now, before the baby comes. Life will be more hectic in four months. We've made a lot of progress on communication skills, but they still need some work.

Josh added,

> Amanda and I have a list of bigger things to keep working on, too—all are "in progress." A major issue is figuring out how Amanda can quit work and stay home once the baby comes. Our initial discussions were a major feat! They included working out the finances, my workload, each of our ability to be with the kids, and so on. We celebrated after talking this through, that's for sure! I'm sure we will have to refine the plan when the baby is actually here.

The couple notes that their communication has improved as they have learned to partner, but they also recognize that there are a few things under the surface that could erupt with the added pressure of a new baby. They have agreed to do one Intentional Dialogue a week for the next month, "even if we have to hire a babysitter so that we can go sit in a coffee shop and have our talk." Josh and Amanda are also committed to including the girls in family meetings. Said Amanda,

> We talk about things we each like and need that week, and the girls really pitch in with their needs as well. They always like to vote on a video or activity. Josh and I then plan our schedules in front of the girls, so everyone is included and they are aware of what's happening. They get to hear us plan our couple time, as well as our individual time with each of them. It helps them understand that we need time together, but we'll give them their special time, too.

## Creating Your Big Picture Date Book

Now it is your turn to create your date book. Because you have been doing the exercises each week and actively working toward your goals together, creating your Big Picture date book should be quite simple. Here are the steps:

Individually, each of you should review all the goals you set together in Step 8, and then review the progress you have made toward these goals in Steps 9 and 10.

Now, each of you should make three lists:

- Issues still unresolved

- Daily details not yet in progress

- Future goals you both have decided to work on within the year

Be sure to include everything on your Individual, Partnership, and Family goals lists. Note the things you have integrated and plan to continue, such as regularly talking and listening and keeping a positive feeling between you.

Next, still working individually, prioritize your goals from most important to least important in your life right now. Indicate which things you need to work on daily, weekly, monthly, semiannually, and annually. Lastly, identify those things that involve your entire family.

Now, come together as partners to discuss your goals for the coming three to four months. Use mirroring and active listening to clarify what each of you desires. Then make a master list of mutually agreed upon Individual, Partnership, and Family goals that are appropriate at this time. Put everything that you are not able to address currently on a list for the future.

Once you have agreed upon the Individual, Partnership, and Family goals you are going to work on in the coming three to four months, schedule conversations, dialogues, and meetings to accomplish your goals. Put these in your Big Picture date book. As before, agree to be accountable and follow through.

## Maintaining Your Progress

Every relationship is different, and every couple has different needs and concerns. The Big Picture approach is meant to be customized according to your unique needs. I encourage you to similarly customize your Big Picture date book, using the following suggestions. You will know which things you need to emphasize and those you already do well:

## Daily

- Maintain ongoing, respectful communication.

- Maintain positive feelings between you.

- Take time to appreciate each other and recognize your mutual resources.

## Each Week

- Schedule regular talking time every other day or four times a week; take turns talking and listening.

- Schedule social time together with others, depending on your needs that week.

- Schedule a weekly partnering meeting and/or family meeting followed by a fun activity or event.

## Biweekly and Monthly

- Schedule a partnering meeting to work on each goal established in Step 8 (and each new goal that you establish). Incorporate dialogue to discuss big issues, plan a new project, or work toward future dreams. As you add new goals and create new action steps, keep track of your "to do" lists; report back on your accomplishments.

- Schedule a monthly financial meeting (to deal with finances— discuss bills, review financial needs and planning, maintain financial health).

- Schedule discussions of topics that you have agreed on, such as Warren and Reba's need to "give back to the world" when they retire, or Amanda and Josh's need to practice the Intentional Dialogue.

## Quarterly

- Review your list of accomplishments and goals.

- Reevaluate and revise for the coming months.

- Celebrate your accomplishments!

- Review your daily details and goal-setting schedule. Delete those goals and action steps that have been completed and integrate new goals and action steps.

## Semiannually or Annually

- Revisit your commitment to each other and to partnering; acknowledge how far you have come.

- Reconsider your values and priorities; update them if necessary.

- Assess your short list of basic partnership needs and make sure you are addressing the ones that are relevant at the time. For example,

| | |
|---|---|
| Household | Social |
| Financial | Sexual |
| Parenting | Spiritual |
| Work | Vacation, play |
| Intellectual pursuits | Others you agree upon |

- Introduce a longer-term goal and make it manageable by breaking it into smaller, doable action steps. Integrate these steps into your date book for the coming months.

## A Master Plan for Living the Partnership of Your Dreams

Big Picture Partnership is a journey, and your Big Picture date book represents your map. Scheduling your regular touchstones together will help you to clearly envision and evaluate where you are headed. It will also keep you on track so that neither of you loses your bearings.

Once these practices and routines become second nature, you'll be a well-seasoned traveler who no longer needs a map. And you'll discover that you and your partner have the energy and time to enjoy each other to the fullest—and to create the ideal life you have envisioned together.

## Some Final Words of Encouragement and Joy

This is the point in most self-help books at which authors wish their readers bon voyage, Godspeed, and good luck. Not me. That doesn't seem like enough. You can't see me from where you are, so I want you to imagine me on the porch of my home, near a city lake. I'm laughing and smiling with delight as I prepare a toast. Here's what I want the two of you to know: I'm not going to wish you a polite, cursory bon voyage, because you're not just beginning your journey now. You and your partner started it long ago, when you first opened this book. And it's not some little journey across town. When you began this program, you took off on a bold, adventurous around-the-world cruise together. It's the trip of a lifetime, and if you were to ever stop, you'd have all kinds of wonderful stories to tell each other.

Only you're not going to stop. If you keep practicing what you've learned here, you'll be living stories of wonder and awe and delight together month after month, year after year, and decade after decade. I'm smiling because I'm filled with excitement for you. Because you're one of those rare couples that genuinely wants to achieve all the promise and joy that you are capable of bringing to each other. It makes me delighted to see two people committed to achieving great happiness and satisfaction together.

So, forget politeness and pallid good wishes. Here's my toast:

*Dare to be great together, to fulfill your mission together, and to achieve your wildest dreams as a couple. Sail on together—each of you with one hand on the wheel, and one arm wrapped tightly around the other's waist. If you look closely, you can see me on my porch, waving and cheering you on.*

# Chapter Notes

## Chapter 3

The 5-to-1 positive-to-negative ratio of interactions comes from the research of John Gottman, PhD. In various discussions of his findings, estimates predicting marital longevity range from 83–94%. See Sally MacDonald, "The State of Marriage in the 90s," *Seattle Times* (July 21, 1996); and John Mordecai Gottman, PhD and Robert Wayne Levenson, PhD, "Rebound from Marital Conflict and Divorce Population," *Family Process*, vol. 38, no. 3 (1999): pp 287–292. Dr. Gottman has published many books on his research that are useful for marriage educators and couples, all of which are recommended to the reader. Among them is the popular *Why Marriages Succeed or Fail and How You Can Make Yours Last*, by John M. Gottman, PhD, and Nan Silver, Fireside: New York, 1995.

## Chapter 5

The parent/adult/child model comes out of Transactional Analysis (TA) which is a social psychology developed by Eric Berne, MD. Over the past forty years the theory has been adopted for use in many fields including psychotherapy, counseling, education, and organizational development. A major text from TA is *I'm OK–You're OK*, by Thomas Harris, PhD. Reissued by Avon: New York, 1993.

For further information on healthy adult development the author recommends the reader to Erik Erickson's social theory of psychology, Abraham Maslow's hierarchy of needs, and any of the following authors and the full range of their book titles. Included here are just a few:

Goleman, Daniel. *Emotional Intelligence: Why it Can Matter More than IQ*. Bantam: New York, 1997.

Seligman, Martin E., PhD. *Authentic Happiness: Using New Positive Psychology to Realize Your Potential for Lasting Fulfillment*. Free Press: New York, 2002.

Sheehy, Gail. *New Passages: Mapping Your Life Across Time*. Random House: New York, 1995.

Sheehy, Gail. *Understanding Men's Passages: Discovering the New Map of Men's Lives*. Ballantine: New York, 1999.

Vaillant, George E. *Aging Well: Surprising Guideposts to a Happier Life from the Landmark Harvard Study of Adult Development*. Little, Brown: New York, 2003.

## Chapter 6

A wide variety of resources cite divorce for marrieds and break-up of those who co-habit around 50% for marrieds and higher for those who cohabit. Some of this is found in documentation from the Rutgers' National Marriage Project, Census Bureau statistics, articles and communications with Mike McManus of Marriage Savers, www.marriagesavers.com, and Dr. Neil Warren.

The National Marriage Project at Rutgers University (www.marriage.rutgers.edu) has a variety of publications detailing recent statistics on marriage, divorce, cohabitation, fertility and childrearing. The "2007 State of Our Unions: The Future of Marriage in America" and the follow-up "2008 Update to the State of Our Unions: Social Indicators Graphs and Tables" provide a thorough overview of marriages at this time.

A classic discussion of long-term love and commitment is found in M. Scott Peck's book *The Road Less Traveled, 25th Anniversary Edition: A New Psychology of Love, Traditional Values and Spiritual Growth*. Touchstone: New York, 2003.

Another useful resource for couples and clients is a 24-page pamphlet entitled, "Intimacy," by Marilyn Mason, PhD, L.C.P., Hazelden: Center City, MN, 1986.

## Chapter 7

The concept of 100% involvement on the part of each partner, and win/win solutions is drawn from the work of Gay and Kathlyn Hendricks, especially their early work, *Conscious Loving: The Journey to Co-Commitment*. Bantam: New York, 1992.

## Chapter 8

Discussion about the ability to resolve conflicts comes from John Gottman, P.D. Dr. Gottman also endorses calming methods when a couple is in the midst of a conflict. He refers to this as "gentle de-escalation and soothing," that are better methods than active listening techniques or mirroring when a couple is in the midst of a conflict. This specific sources comes from a 1999 Futurist article entitled "Predicting Successful Marriages," (Cynthia G. Wagner, vol. 33, no. 6, June/July 1999), received from Dr. Gottman's office.

Additional studies and clinical applications on the topic of conflict resolution include work by Clifford Notarius, Scott Stanley, and Howard Markman. Some additional titles include:

Markman, Howard, Scott Stanley, and Susan L. Blumberg. *Fighting for Your Marriage: Positive Steps for Preventing Divorce and Preserving a Lasting Love*. Jossey-Bass: San Francisco, 2001.

Notarius, Clifford, Clifford Notarius I., and Howard Markman, ed. *We Can Work It Out: How to Solve Conflicts, Save Your Marriage, and Strengthen Your Love for Each Other*. Perigee: New York, 1994.

Drs. John and Julie Gottman conduct couples workshops throughout the year in Seattle, Washington. During the workshop, couples gain new insights and learn research-based relationship skills that can improve the intimacy and friendship in their relationship. More information can be found at their Web site www.gottman.com.

One of the most successful programs for couples in trouble is PREP: The Prevention and Relationship Enhancement Program, founded and directed by Howard Markman, PhD, and Scott Stanley, PhD. PREP is based on over twenty years of research and can be found online at www.prepinc.com.

## Chapter 9

The full reference for Eileen McCann's book, enthusiastically mentioned in this chapter is: McCann, Eileen. *The Two-Step: The Dance Toward Intimacy.* Grove Press: New York, 1987.

## Chapter 11

The intentional dialogue is taken directly from the work of Harville Hendrix. Various versions of the dialogue process can be found online at a number of Imago Therapy Web sites, however the version utilized in this book is a translation, from the author's experience in a workshop with Harville Hendrix himself. Dr. Hendrix's best-known work is *Getting the Love You Want: A Guide For Couples.* Owl Books: New York, 2001.

For additional resources a program that teaches mediation, negotiation, and communication skills is offered through Harvard University's Law School. Readable books from the Harvard program include:

Fisher, Roger, and Scott Brown. *Getting Together: Building Relationships as We Negotiate.* Penguin: New York, 1989.

Fisher, Roger, Bruce Patten, and William Ury. *Getting to Yes: Negotiating Agreement Without Giving In.* 2nd ed. Penguin: New York, 1991.

Ury, William. *Getting Past No: Negotiating in Difficult Situations.* Revised ed. Bantam: New York, 1993.

## Chapter 12

There are a wide variety of creativity resources available on the bookshelves and online. For initial grounding in this topic, the author highly recommends the following resources:

Bepko, Claudia, and Jo-Ann Krestan. *Singing at the Top of Our Lungs: Women, Love, and Creativity.* HarperCollins: New York, 1993.

Cameron, Julia. *The Artist's Way: A Spiritual Path to Higher Creativity.* Putnam: New York, 1992.

Czikszentmihalyi, Mihaly. *Creativity: Flow and the Psychology of Discovery and Invention.* HarperCollins: New York, 1997.

Czikszentmihalyi, Mihaly. *Flow: The Psychology of Optimal Experience.* HarperCollins: New York, 1990.

Fritz, Robert. *Creating.* Ballantine: New York, 1993.

Fritz, Robert. *The Path of Least Resistance: Learning to Become the Creative Force in Your Own Life.* Revised and expanded. Fawcett Columbine: New York, 1989.

Harman, Willis, PhD, and Howard Rheingold. *Higher Creativity: Liberating the Unconscious for Breakthrough Insights.* Tarcher: New York, 1984.

# Resources

## Smart Marriages

One of the main resources for both couples and marriage education professionals is The Coalition for Marriage, Couples, and Family Education, LLC. This comprehensive and free service can be viewed online at www. smartmarriages.com.

Smart Marriages exists for the betterment and promotion of research, education, legislation, and support of healthy relationships. You can receive an informative online newsletter, use the extensive directory to look up a class or workshop anywhere in the world, and become connected to the very latest research, books, and resources available through this resource.

Smart Marriages also provides an annual conference each summer where upwards of 2,500 people gather from all over the nation, and the world, to discuss, promote, become informed about, and celebrate healthy marriage. This low-cost, annual event provides great opportunity to network with other couples, marriage educators, peer mentors, and a wide variety of other experts in an informal atmosphere. The format involves pre- and post-training Institutes for couples and educators, a wide variety of exhibitors, lunch and dinner presentations by leaders in the field, and a large number of informative workshops throughout the entire three-day conference itself.

## The National Marriage Project

This initiative, located at Rutgers University, is co-directed by two leading family experts and well-known authors, David Popenoe, PhD, and Barbara Dafoe Whitehead, PhD. Its mission is to strengthen the institution of marriage by providing research that informs public policy, educates the public, and focuses attention on the consequences of problems in marriage on the millions of children in our nation. The National Marriage Project Web site can be viewed online at www.marriage.rutgers.edu. It includes a list of publications and links that are informative and useful.

# Acknowledgments

I would like to acknowledge my primary mentors: the many clients I have worked with over the years. I am always humbled by their tenacity, perseverance, and desire to make their relationships more meaningful, as well as their courage and vulnerability in opening up to me. They have been, and continue to be, my greatest teachers.

I am also grateful for the community of literary consultants and editors who helped shape earlier versions of this book. They gave me their unwavering support along with insightful editorial suggestions. These include Paulette Bates-Alden, Scott Edelstein, Laura Golden Bellotti, and Judy Arginteanu. Meredith Hale and her staff at Sterling Publishing have been a delight to work with as they shepherd this project to market. Finally, I am indebted to Joy Tutela my agent at David Black Literary Agency. She saw how important this book was right from the start. Thanks to you all.

# Index